UNDERSTANDING
CANCER

A PRACTICAL GUIDE FOR PATIENTS AND FAMILIES:

Causes, Treatment Options, Prevention, and Emotional Support

Nhon Charles Ntungwe

Disclaimer:

This book is intended for informational and educational purposes only. It is not intended to provide medical advice, diagnosis, or treatment recommendations. The content is not a substitute for professional medical advice, consultation, diagnosis, or treatment from a qualified healthcare provider. Always seek the advice of your physician or other qualified health professionals with any questions you may have regarding a medical condition. The author and publisher disclaim any liability for the use or misuse of the information contained in this book.

TABLE OF CONTENTS

Preface

Understanding Cancer is a document that has been properly researched and is explicit to the ordinary or lay person who does not have a medical background. Most of the topics discussed in this book were selected by my former patients. Some of these patients happen to be healthcare professionals, including doctors. No doctor can treat all forms of cancer, so this guide is primarily to help patients understand what options are available to guide their decision-making in seeking cancer care.

With cancer emerging as one of the deadliest diseases in human history, the world needs to be educated on the rapid advancements in technology and research. Considering this trend, Understanding Cancer will contribute to and enhance your knowledge about the available options regarding cancer care. Do yourself, your family, and your friends a favor and peace of mind by getting a copy.

Nhon Charles M Ntungwe BS RT(R)(T)
Founder, Global Cancer Consultants
Executive Director, Afric-med USA

Acknowledgments

To my wife, Gwendoline Epie Ntungwe, who is always there for me, thank you for your continued support. To our two children, Lauren Ebude and Hayden Kome, who always laugh at me for my failed ventures. You two are a force for my inspiration.

To my parents Ferdinand Ntungwe Ngunde and Hannah Dione. Thank you, Dad, for believing in me even when I failed an exam. To my friends, Nzene Sylvester Enongene, Valentine Nkowa Sr., and my teacher at Howard University and Georgetown, Professor Lloyd Campbell.

To Dr. Ivo Nnane, who was the first person to critique my work. My appreciation to Dr. Maceline Yaya for correcting my work. To my cousin, Divisional Police Commissioner Vincent Etue Mbulle, who helped me come to America when he was First Secretary at the Embassy of Cameroon in Washington, DC. I love you all.

Much gratitude goes to my patients, especially those at the National Institute of Health (NIH) and Georgetown University Hospital. Thank you all so much. Your concerns, questions, and experiences inspired me to write this book.

Introduction

If either you or someone close to you has been diagnosed with cancer, you will realize that you have become an actor on stage. Cancer happens to be one of those rare diseases that involve many actors at one point or another. That is why it is important to know at which point you must come in.

It is important to understand that there are more than one hundred forms of cancer out there. It is equally imperative for patients and their families to know that no single cancer doctor can treat all forms of cancer. It is equally good to know that even if two patients have the same type of cancer, form, and or stage, for example, breast cancer, the treatment approaches might never be the same.

Having this in mind, the purpose of *A Practical Approach Cancer Prevention and Treatment* is to act as a reference for some causes, prevention, treatment, and recovery methods for cancer patients.

CHAPTER 1
What is cancer?

The number of patients diagnosed with cancer increases year after year. As defined by the American Cancer Society, this is a disease in which abnormal cells divide uncontrollably and destroy body tissues. The lives of those diagnosed with cancer are turned upside down in an instant. Concerns, worries, and plans regarding every aspect of life, which include but are not limited to relationships, work, pleasure, money, treatment, and transportation, all come into play. But the most difficult question that the patient has, which always supersedes the rest and is never spoken of, is whether I am going to die. Not necessarily; it is not like a car or airplane accident, whereby there might be no survivors. Being diagnosed with cancer is not the end of the world, as some patients claim it to be, though a patient always thinks so, especially with the stigma attached to the disease. I have heard some patients say they prefer to be diagnosed with HIV/AIDS instead of cancer. Why so, I ask? Because of the advancement in medicine, AIDS patients can now live longer.

Considerable progress has now been made in the treatment of cancer. Some of these treatments are curative, and non-curative treatments can lengthen and improve the quality of life. Although the stage at which a cancer is diagnosed might determine if it can be cured, the following cancers have a high probability of being cured. They include testicular cancer, breast cancer, osteogenic sarcoma, Hodgkin's disease, Wilms' tumor, which is kidney cancer in children, prostate cancer, some forms of muscle cancer (rhabdomyosarcoma), and gynecological cancer. (In a book titled *Informed Decisions: The Complete Book of Cancer Diagnosis, Treatment, and Recovery*, co-authored by Gerald P. Murphy, M.D., Lois B. Morris, and Dianne Lange, 1997).

CAUSES OF CANCER

Scientists have been working very hard to determine the cause of cancer. It is, therefore, not possible to know the exact cause of cancer between two people who might have the same form of the disease. The question that puzzles physicians, academia, and even ordinary people is what made it happen. Though the research process regarding the causes of cancer continues, certain risk factors have been identified so far. On the other hand, there are equally other factors known as protective factors, which lower the risk of developing some forms of cancer.

Exposure to some substances and or chemicals, as well as some behaviors such as oral sex, poses a risk of contracting head and neck cancer (HPV), huge alcohol consumption, diet (fat), hormones, infectious agents, obesity, tobacco use, sunlight, and occupations such as mining and petroleum are prone to causing lung cancers, environment, etc. There are equally some uncontrollable factors like hereditary (genes) as well as aging. A family history of cancer is a risk factor, indicating that members of that family might eventually develop that type of cancer. Breast, colon, and rectal cancers are very high in this category (NCI, 2022).

Most scientists and writers will categorize risk factors as major and minor. But from experience, every risk factor should be given maximum consideration and or attention, and your chances of contracting one form of cancer or the other will be minimized.

Alcohol

Alcohol consumption is one of the major risk factors, though it sometimes works in partnership with tobacco. The probability of heavy drinkers developing mouth, head and neck or liver cancers is very high. Although the evidence for the linkage between breast cancer and alcohol is low, heavy drinking is more often associated with cirrhosis, which causes changes in liver tissues and eventually leads to liver cancer. However, even in the absence of alcohol being a causative factor, liver cancer can still develop. An unusual case of a seven-year-old liver cancer case was recently treated with proton therapy at Georgetown University Hospital in Washington, DC.

Tobacco

Tobacco use is probably the greatest risk factor as far as cancer causes are concerned. Lung cancer is linked to high tobacco use. It is equally evident that heavy smokers are, in most cases, heavy drinkers as well. Cancers of the lung, bladder, pancreas, head and neck, and kidney, in most cases, have a direct association with tobacco use (Murphy, G.P., Morris, L.B., & Lange, D., 1997). The circulation of smoke from the airways to other parts of the body increases the chances of developing some of the above-mentioned cancers, which are distanced from the lungs.

Tobacco use is not limited only to cigarette smokers. Chewing tobacco, though to a lesser extent, is equally risky. Secondhand smoke is a contributing factor, too. This occurs through inhalation from cigarettes or cigars without direct smoke from the individual.

Smokeless tobacco products are known to contain some potentially harmful chemicals, like polonium. These carcinogens are absorbed through the mouth, and this might be one of the reasons why many cancers are linked to smokeless tobacco. Smokeless tobacco products, on average, are known to cause less cancer than cigarettes. Again, though they are being promoted as less harmful than cigarettes, they are also a product to be concerned with.

Indirectly, radioactive materials that are transmitted into tobacco leaves used to make cigarettes or cigars are equally linked to cancer causes. These materials come from the fertilizer and soil used to grow tobacco leaves. The amount in the tobacco will, therefore, depend on the soil the plants were grown on and the type of fertilizer used. These radioactive materials are given up as smoke and inhaled when tobacco is burned, which, of course, might lead to lung cancer (ACS, 2019).

Diet

The type and nature of food consumed have become one of those risk factors that are attracting much attention nowadays. The number of deaths caused by cancer that occur because of diet is on the rise. This is associated with the type of foods, methods of preparation, portions, varieties, and calorie balance.

Fatty diets have been associated with some forms of cancer, such as prostate, colon, endometrial, and rectum. Some theories equally associate breast cancer with a high-fat diet, but this link is weak. Studies have shown that more Western countries with a fatty diet are associated with the above-mentioned cancers than a country like Japan, which has a higher fiber and lower fat consumption rate (ACS, 2019). Fiber plays a preventive role in some, as far as some of these fatty foods are concerned. Insoluble fiber is thought to reduce the risk of colon cancer. Heavy weight or obesity, which is a result of heavy eating, is also a risk factor for many types of cancers, like breast, prostate, and rectum.

The American Cancer Society recommends eating fewer fatty foods and more fiber-rich foods and vegetables. Certain ways of food preparation and additives are also risk factors. For example, smoked foods cause stomach cancer. The American Cancer Society's nutritional guidelines advise the consumption of high proportions of plant foods such as fruits, vegetables, grains, and beans. It equally recommends limited amounts of meat, dairy, and other high-fat foods and more physical activities.

Custom, Sex, and Reproductive Behaviors

Backgrounds and choices are sometimes risk factors for the cause of certain cancers. This might affect the individuals personally, their families, or their children. For example, male children who are circumcised reduce the risk of having cancer for themselves and their future partners. The female partners of circumcised males have a lower risk of cervical cancer than those whose partners are uncircumcised. This could be due to Human Papillomavirus (HPV) or poor hygiene.

Late childbearing in women increases the risk of breast cancer as well. It is equally believed that avoiding childbirth in women might be linked to breast cancer. Promiscuity, which is the behavior of having multiple sex partners, exposes a female to sexually transmitted diseases like HPV, which eventually leads to cervical cancer.

Infectious Agents

Some infectious agents, through viruses, are linked to certain types of cancers. This is because viruses can invade cells, which eventually can cause cancer. The Epstein-Barr virus is associated with Burkitt's lymphoma. Burkett's lymphoma is a tumor found in children, mostly in Africa. HPV, which causes genital warts, also causes cervical cancer (ACS, 2019). The chances of developing head and neck cancers from HPV due to oral sex habits cannot be ruled out. HPV enters the body when one performs vaginal, anal, or oral sex with someone who has the virus. Cancers caused by this virus are sometimes difficult to detect because they do not show any symptoms.

The hepatitis B virus is a well-known virus that causes liver cancer all over the world. It is equally noted that the acquired immune deficiency syndrome (AIDS) virus is connected to Kaposi's sarcoma and some lymphomas. A type of leukemia mostly found in the Caribbean and Japan is linked to the human T-cell leukemia virus.

Hereditary

The fact that you are born into certain families makes you prone to having some cancers. Some of these cancers include but are not limited to, breast cancer, colon cancer, ovarian cancer, etc. The recurrence rate is generation after generation. It is, therefore, important to know your family medical history because some of these cancers can be prevented with constant checkups. For instance, breast self-examination and mammograms can lead to early detection of breast cancer, colonoscopy for colon cancer, and Pap smear for gynecological cancer. The importance of knowing your family medical history should not be underestimated.

Medical Treatments

Some recommended treatment modalities themselves can cause cancer. Some drugs used in chemotherapy, which are meant to fight cancer, can sometimes be carcinogenic. Immunosuppressant drugs used in conjunction with organ transplants reduce the body's ability to fight malignancies. Much accumulated radiation from diagnostic X-rays and radiation therapy can cause cancer as well.

7

Environment and Hazards

Hazards such as atomic bombs in Hiroshima, radiation in Chernobyl, and the recent military explosion in Russia are cancer-prone. Some homes and buildings also contain some amount of unknown radiation. Sunlight or ultraviolet radiation equally poses a risk, especially to the light-skinned population. Air pollution and asbestos from chemicals, mining, and petroleum industries are all cancer-prone hazards. Some people who have lived in Camp Lejeune are known to have been prone to cancer because of the environment and water contamination.

Occupational Causes

Certain occupations have been identified as exposing workers to carcinogens. In a nutshell, people in certain professions are at risk of developing cancer. These include workers in mining, chemicals, rubber, manufacturing, agriculture, industrial materials, petroleum, dyes, dust, lead, etc. Healthcare professionals exposed to diagnostic X-rays, radon, or other forms of ionizing radiation are also at risk of developing cancer.

CHAPTER 2
Treatment

It is always bad news for everybody, including doctors and other healthcare providers, if diagnosed with cancer. The most important aspect of the cancer treatment process is seeking a second opinion. There are tons of cancer doctors out there, but as a layperson, you will be surprised to know that there is no single doctor who can treat all forms of cancer correctly. Secondly, it is equally very important to visit another clinic to make sure what information is given to you by one facility or claim you have is the disease you have been diagnosed with. Some studies have shown that there are false positives as well as malpractices going on all over the world. As a patient or a relative of a patient, you must make sure the diagnoses you are given are what you have.

Treatment team

Cancer is not a one-size-fits-all professional approach. It requires a team of healthcare professionals throughout a patient's treatment journey and after. Developing a treatment plan is complex because you will need the advice and recommendations of many professionals. Nowadays, lots of cancer centers have a team available to help navigate the process. The American Cancer Society has also done a good job in this regard. Depending on your diagnosis and stage of cancer, the list of healthcare professionals below is among those who will work with you and your family in the treatment journey.

Primary Care Doctor

Your primary care doctor or personal physician is always your main point of contact. After your diagnosis, your primary care doctor will refer you to a cancer doctor who specializes in your type of cancer or disease. It is equally important to seek a second opinion away from your referred cancer doctor to select or make a comfortable choice.

Surgeon

The surgeon is a doctor who specializes in surgery. These are doctors who undergo additional training after medical school to perform surgery or to operate on human beings. Do not hesitate to Google or ask questions about your surgeon. Remember, it is your body and not anyone else's.

Medical Oncologist

A medical oncologist is a cancer doctor who prescribes and administers cancer drugs or chemotherapy. This physician undergoes additional training after medical school and becomes board-certified. Chemotherapy is, in most cases, administered intravenously; that is, it is injected slowly into the bloodstream through the vein in a hospital setting, and the patient is observed in case of any reactions.

Radiation Oncologist

The radiation oncologist is the cancer doctor who uses radiation to treat your cancer. This specialist doctor undergoes further training or residency to specialize in this type of practice. Not all radiation oncologists or cancer doctors might be proficient in your type of cancer. Always get a track record of your recommended physician.

Pathologist

The pathologist is the doctor who examines the tissues or body parts removed from a patient. This doctor also stages and classifies the cancer, and based on the pathological results, a recommendation on a treatment plan is made. In most cases, though, based on a patient's staging, the most popular recommended treatment plans are surgery, chemotherapy, and radiation therapy.

Radiation Therapist

Radiation therapists are professionals who work under the radiation oncologist to administer the radiation to the patient as prescribed by the radiation oncologist. These are board-certified personnel after their college education. Your radiation therapist is the professional who will be administering your radiation daily. This individual is one of your best friends during your entire treatment period because sometimes the treatment is as long as six weeks. The radiation therapist will be able to answer most of your questions and or concerns or refer the patient to the nurse, doctor, or social worker, in a nutshell, the people you might not have daily access to.

Nurse Navigator

The nurse navigator is a nurse who specializes in cancer care or oncology. The nurse navigator can help the patient with additional resources they might need, such as transportation in and out of treatment facilities, physical therapy, appointments, and insurance issues.

Social Worker

A social worker is a trained professional who helps a patient with logistics. This includes meals, pastoral care, wills, legal advice, etc.

TREATMENT OPTIONS

Selecting treatment options for your cancer is a very crucial decision for your well-being, both during and after treatment. There have been reoccurrences because of poor treatment or mismanagement of the disease. There have also been situations of metastases, a situation whereby cancer spreads to other parts of the body, sometimes because of poor treatment. Based on the stage of the disease, the approaches will either be palliative, curative, or radical.

Curative or radical treatment aims to cure the disease. This mode of treatment is chosen after the pathological results have indicated that the cancer is localized. Palliative treatment, on the other hand, aims to treat symptoms or reduce pain. This might be because the cancer has spread to other parts of the body or metastasized. To accomplish any of the above objectives, the physician will now choose any or a combination of the following options.

Surgery

Surgery is the act of removing tissues and their surroundings for either diagnosis or treatment. In this context, if a patient has been diagnosed with cancer, the tumor will be removed by surgery, and a pathologist will also examine the surrounding cells to make sure residues are not left behind. In most cases, surgery goes hand in hand with another mode of treatment, such as chemotherapy, radiation therapy, or the three.

Chemotherapy

Chemotherapy is a mode of treatment whereby a cancer drug is either injected into the bloodstream or taken by mouth and circulated around the body to kill cancer cells. Chemotherapy either helps to kill cancer cells or helps to shrink the tumor. It is not unusual to combine chemotherapy and radiation therapy to treat cancer. That is, taking both types of therapies concordantly. Some of the side effects of chemo include nausea, vomiting, weight loss, loss of appetite, and hair loss. Hair loss is the side effect that always concerns most patients. Yes, a patient will lose their hair, but it will always grow back to normal. This and other concerns should always be addressed by the doctor or the healthcare professional who is taking care of the patient.

Questions for your Doctor

- Will I lose my hair from getting chemotherapy?

- What are the side effects of this type of treatment?

- In case I can't eat real food, what is my next best alternative?

- Will this affect my thinking or reasoning ability?

- Will I have neuropathy because I am diabetic, and if so, how can I prevent it?

- Can I take a flu vaccine before my chemotherapy treatment for fear of flu or my immune system being compromised?

Immunotherapy

Immunotherapy is one of those forms of biological therapy that is very popular in cancer treatment. Another form of body therapy is cytotoxic therapy. Cytotoxic therapy is an approach where proteins called cytotoxins are produced by the body cells to attack the cancer cells or make them difficult to grow or reproduce (Murphy, G.P., Morris, L.B., & Lange, D., 1997).

Most scientists might say that passive immunotherapy may prove to be the best form of biological therapy. With this strategy, antibodies and other agents that have been activated in the lab are given to patients with cancer. Another name for this approach is adoptive immunotherapy because the person adopts an immune response that has been developed in the test tube. This approach might require a long hospital stay, be expensive, and require close monitoring of the patient.

Bone Marrow Transplant

A bone marrow transplant is the removal of bone marrow from one person and the return of blood-forming cells later to the same person or the transfer of blood-forming cells to someone else. Though a bone marrow transplant might be good for other medical purposes, such as aplastic anemia, most of the transplants performed today are to help treat cancer. This mode of treatment is not always a treatment in itself, as most people think, but it allows patients with cancer to undergo very aggressive therapy.

Clinical Trials

Studies involving humans are crucial to treating or conquering cancer. These investigational aspects of medicine have led to a progressive understanding of the disease for diagnoses, prevention, and treatment. Clinical trials are approved by the American Cancer Society, oncologists, and the National Cancer Institute. Since cancer medicine is always updated as to what is new in the market, patients who undergo clinical trials are exposed to treatments that, in most cases, are not even on the market or in circulation yet. The rate of cancer patients who volunteer for clinical trials is basic, but scientists believe that if they had more volunteers, it would be better for medicine.

In most cases, patients have the impression that if they are undergoing clinical trials, they may be treated as guinea pigs.

Scientists and oncologists have noted this fear. These trials are not undertaken by a single doctor but by a group of physicians. The downside of this practice is that since clinical trials are still in a progressive stage, the side effects are not all known yet.

Information on Clinical Trials

While most clinical trials or studies on cancer are carried out by universities, research institutions, and hospitals alongside associated clinics, the funding is mostly provided by the National Cancer Institute. To minimize patient movements, primary care doctors link with oncologists through the Community Clinical Trial Oncology Program (CCOP). This ensures that patients don't have to leave their primary areas if possible. It is not uncommon for pharmaceutical companies to work with research and cancer centers on clinical trials, especially if they want to prove the effectiveness of their medicine or treatment. But the scientific rules are strict, and everybody or company follows the same rules.

Normally, there are many ways to go about finding out about clinical trials that may benefit you. Though your primary care doctor can be of great use, the most obvious sources will be your oncologist and the National Cancer Institute (NCI, 2022). The Cancer Information Service, a program supported by NCI, will be another source of helpful contact information for physicians in their database for various diseases. NCI is equally in collaboration with some advocacy organizations like the National Alliance of Breast Cancer Organizations to offer information about clinical trials through their websites. Generally, patient advocacy groups are good sources of experimental treatment. Like any other form of treatment, always ask questions. Some of these questions will be listed later in the book.

Questions for your Doctor

- What is my next best alternative if this clinical trial doesn't work?

- Has this type of treatment been tested on humans before?

- Where can I get more information on this type of study?

- Can you connect me to other people who have had clinical trials before?

- What is the worst-case scenario for this type of treatment?

- How soon can I get help if I have adverse side effects or reactions from this type of treatment?

Radiation Therapy

The use of high-energy X-rays in cancer treatment is known as radiation therapy or radiotherapy. Most cancer patients will use this form of treatment, which is either used alone or alongside other forms of treatment such as surgery and chemotherapy. This treatment method works by damaging genetic materials within the cell, thus making it difficult for them to divide. During radiation therapy treatment, both normal and cancer cells are affected. But while the normal cells regenerate, the cancer cells die. Radiation therapy treats only a localized area where there is cancer. However, total body radiation might be recommended for some patients who are undergoing other forms of treatment, such as bone marrow transplantation. Depending on the area to be treated using radiation, patients of childbearing age or who wish to have babies after radiation should have a conversation with their doctor or the radiation oncologist during consultation before treatment begins. There are usually pre-treatment consultations or procedures, sometimes within the same establishment or referrals made. Hair loss is usually one of the greatest patients' concerns when they are about to undergo radiation therapy. Normally, only the treatment area is affected, except when a patient is receiving another form of treatment, such as chemotherapy.

Radiation therapy is administered only in specialized hospitals by a team of specialists headed by a radiation doctor known as a radiation oncologist. Always have a conversation with your oncologist about the possible side effects of the radiation and or other forms of treatment.

Questions for Your Cancer Doctor

- What type of treatment am I having?

- Can you explain to me why I am having this type of treatment for my cancer?

- What could be my next best alternative?

- What reactions or side effects should I expect from this type of treatment?

- What will this treatment do for my disease? Is it going to shrink or eliminate my tumor?

- How and when do I find out if the treatment is working?

- How many patients have you treated who have the same disease, and what has been the outcome?

CHAPTER 3
Alternative and Complementary Therapies

Conventional cancer treatment options, which include surgery, chemotherapy, and radiation therapy, are usually very effective methods of treatment, and their successes have been scientifically proven. While researching your options as a patient, you will come across or hear about other options, such as a special diet, acupuncture, new compounds, traditional or herbal medicine, etc. Some of these other aspects may be incorporated into your treatment, but some might be harmful.

Again, when weighing your options for managing your disease, conventional treatment methods, as mentioned earlier, have been proven by Western scientists to be very effective. Alternative medicine, by contrast, might not have been evaluated effectively. There are many such alternatives.

Meditation

Meditation is one of the many ways to relax, and some claim it can cure cancer. Some studies have proven that it can relieve pain, nausea, and other uncomfortable side effects of cancer treatment. Other studies have shown that meditation and relaxation can decrease blood pressure, respiratory rate, and metabolism, which all contribute to reducing stress.

Meditation can be practiced in many ways, such as focusing on a repeated word, concentrating on an object, such as a bird building its nest, sitting quietly, and concentrating on a regular breathing pattern. Some forms of yoga, such as hatha yoga, can also help to reduce stress and anxiety.

Acupuncture

Acupuncture is the process of inserting extremely fine needles into points along meridians called acupoints and pressing on them. It is believed to enhance the flow of energy to the corresponding organs and systems. Though practiced all over the world, acupuncture has its origin in China. Current research suggests that acupuncture may work by triggering the release of natural pain inhibitors. Though it has not been proven to treat cancer directly, it helps to relieve pain from the disease.

Herbal Treatment

Cancer is an old disease, and more than four thousand plants have reportedly been used to treat it worldwide. Though herbal treatment in the Western world is mostly based on Chinese medicine, other parts of the world, like Africa, are equally practicing this form of treatment. While some herbs are used alone as tea, others can be a combination of teas.

Nutritional Therapy

From experience, cancer affects one's nutritional needs in many ways. Diet professionals or nutritionists will design an eating plan for a cancer patient, taking into consideration the likes and dislikes of the individual as well as the type of cancer, area of treatment, and treatment type. Foods are chosen to help improve well-being, quality of life, and tolerance to your cancer treatment. Weight loss is a big factor of concern for patients who are undergoing cancer treatment. A nutritionist takes into consideration the number of calories, balance, moderation, and variety to keep a patient's weight from falling drastically, thus preventing any danger that may arise from this downturn. Nutritionists and oncologists will recommend low-fat and high-fiber foods to cancer patients. Studies are still underway to prove that this recommendation might prevent a recurrence of a properly treated cancer. It has not been proven that either foods or drinks have been able to treat any form of cancer (Be a Survivor 2007, Vladimir Lange, M.D.).

Mind and Body Connection

Sometimes, it is normal and appropriate to experience a range of difficult and mixed feelings throughout your illness and recovery. Some of such experiences include anger, anxiety, depression, guilt, fear, and worry. Anger, fear, etc., seem to have a negative effect on the body. Learning how to cope with all these emotional issues using comprehensive approaches such as spiritual support, participation in support groups, and visualization may benefit your health because it may help speed up the recovery process. Anyone with cancer can benefit from learning emotional regulation skills as well as techniques to cope with all this distress through the thought process and behaviors.

Vitamins and Minerals

A variety of compounds, including certain vitamins and minerals, have been used with various successes to decrease the side effects of cancer treatment. Ewan Cameron, in the 1970s, believed that large doses of vitamin C would help slow down the progression of the disease by increasing the amount of substance in the blood known to inhibit tumor growth and by strengthening the cells around the tumor to make it more resistant to the cancer cells. Some other studies funded by the National Cancer Institute and conducted by the Mayo Clinic did not find any significant improvement in people who took large amounts of vitamin C compared to those who took a placebo. Ask your healthcare provider to review and give you the latest updates in this regard (Informed Decisions, Murphy, G.P., Morris, L.B., & Lange, D., 1997).

Spiritual and Other Support Groups

From experience, even those who have little or no connection with religion often find themselves with cancer emergencies and a feeling of helplessness. Prayers and other forms of spiritual imagery or inner dialogue have helped patients find strength within themselves to cope with cancer or other terminal diseases.

Support groups, according to research and experiences, have shown themselves to be a valuable part of cancer treatment and can have a positive effect on your quality of life and attitude. Experiences have shown that meeting with people who have similar emotional and physical experiences can help eliminate an individual's feelings of isolation. Having a positive attitude toward a friend or relative with cancer is very helpful. Support groups provide an environment where you can express your emotions among sympathizers. Many support groups are run by healthcare professionals and other cancer survivors. These groups can contribute important information on cancer, such as diet and physical and emotional disturbance.

People who join support groups during or after cancer treatment are more likely not only to feel better but also to live longer. Sometimes, recurrences are equally prevented due to shared experiences from other group members. Support groups have conclusively been proven to be beneficial. Some evidence suggests that social and or moral support may have a positive effect on the immune system. Secondly, patients who feel that others care about their well-being are likely to eat well, get enough sleep, take their medication regularly as directed, and meet up with their hospital appointments (ACS, 2019).

Making Choices

It is usually bad news if a person is diagnosed with cancer. Patients often find themselves asking, 'Why me?'. It is, therefore, sometimes very difficult to make an objective decision on the mode of treatment with the hope of a cure. Nevertheless, fear and depression shouldn't impair your judgment. The well-researched modes of treatment, which include surgery, chemotherapy, and radiation therapy, should be your first choice of treatment. Nowadays, there are lots of advertisements all over the various media that are convincing. Again, do not be persuaded to make a decision that might cost you later.

CHAPTER 4
The Pain Episode

An astonishing number of people experience cancer-related pain all over the world daily. The good part about this aspect of the experience is that if it is treatment or therapy-related, you are not the first person to be in that situation. Remedies are usually available.

Experiences have shown that cancer-related pain had not been factored into the quality of care for cancer patients. But as it is with other aspects of cancer care advancement, there has been much improvement in pain management from the disease. To control or manage pain, an aggressive measure is usually implemented either by drugs or surgery to give the maximum relief to the patient. There are also some other techniques to improve quality of life, such as enjoyment of recreation, which might aid you to function as normally as possible, including the ability to work and for self-help in the most extreme situations. Psychological therapy, as well as some other techniques that do not require medication, like yoga, have also been proven to be helpful.

Pain Concept

Pain is a situation whereby something hurts in a part of the body. Pain is transmitted to the brain by thousands of nerves from all parts of the body immediately where harm is incurred. Cancer-related pain, which is our topic of discussion, is most incurred when the disease invades muscles, bones, and or blood vessels. It can also occur if the disease blocks hollow organs, presses on the nerves, or pinches blood vessels. Pain can also be caused by cancer-related treatment itself. A case in point is pain incurred when a patient is undergoing radiation therapy treatment. In some cases, due to excessive pain from body reactions, including some other side effects from the treatment, patients take a break from the treatment for about a week to manage them before returning to their normal treatment course.

Pain is also beyond the physical aspect of the feeling. Usually, the longer the pain, the greater it causes other aspects of human suffering. Uncontrolled or unrelieved pain makes it difficult for the patient to carry out certain activities like eating, walking, dressing oneself, or even taking a bath. This, in some cases, makes a patient angry, anxious, or depressed. This ultimately strips a patient's dignity, and relationships with friends and relatives are shattered. It equally makes the patient start having the impression that the doctors are not doing enough to get their situation under control. There is also much mistrust among other healthcare professionals who are doing their best for a common goal of maximum care. In extreme cases, the patient becomes frustrated and unwilling to comply or continue the prescribed treatment, which might help to alleviate the pain.

What is unique about pain is that it hurts, but the level of pain is different between individuals, backgrounds, or cultures. In hospitals or medical settings, pain ratings are usually from 0 to 10, with 0 being the least pain and 10 being the maximum pain. But these numbers are relative to each individual and sometimes might be misleading. In a nutshell, levels of endurance are different among patients.

It is noted that fear gives a different connotation to pain. Most patients will automatically believe that as soon as they are diagnosed with cancer, they start associating the disease with pain. Though pain is a common complication with certain types of cancers, it is not inevitable that it will occur. On the other hand, even if it does occur, it doesn't mean that it is going to get worse. The treatment for cancer or tumors, in some cases, relieves the pain. In some instances, the pain might get worse as the treatment progresses, but that does not mean that the treatment is not effective or that the cancer might not be cured.

Pain Control

Communication is the first and probably the most important step in the pain relief process. Your doctor or healthcare provider needs to know what is going on with you. Patients must help their doctors help them by giving accurate information concerning their condition. Remember, like cancer, your pain is unique. It is only you who is feeling that pain and nobody else. Below are some strategies that are very helpful to the patient with pain.

Stay on top of the pain by possible anticipation and quick response. The more an individual can prevent pain from developing or becoming severe, the more effective the treatment might be, which might help to lower your doses. Take medications or treatment as prescribed by your healthcare provider.

From experience, most patients will never complain about the pain they have until it becomes unbearable. Do not be afraid to admit you have pain. Communicating with your caregiver or family member is essential, for it is only you who knows how you feel. Patients should not be worried about being seen as complainers or difficult patients. Pain relief is vital as far as managing cancer is concerned, and if someone does not know your situation, including your pain level, they will not be able to give you as much help as you deserve.

Most patients will not follow their doctor's orders. To get the most benefit, a patient might need to take their medication at certain intervals. Equally, speak out if you are getting the relief or not because, based on your level of pain, an additional dose might be required. The effect of cancer on one's body might change from time to time. The medication that might have worked in the past may not be effective for your present condition. Keep in mind that the doctor or healthcare professional is there for you, and always report any side effects and progress to these individuals.

Individual Experience

The patient is the most important individual in the case plan team. The more involved the patient is, the more you will understand the concept and be able to communicate well, and your pain will be brought under control. A couple of factors make the pain experience individualistic. Some patients with cancer may downplay the extent of pain, while others will not want to distract from their primary disease, which is cancer, thus trying to make cancer the priority. It is not uncommon for some patients to fear addiction to pain medications such as narcotics. Some people will want to put forth a brave face to prevent loved ones from knowing the level of their suffering. Again, it is important to let others know about your condition. Do not take this journey alone.

Studies have shown that psychology plays a big role in patients when it comes to pain. Fear and other concerns or worries about a patient's disease can influence pain. Patients who are less worried and have less fear have a higher tolerance level than those who are much more concerned about their pain. The patient with the most worries tends to get less sleep, which might lead to other complications.

Emotional problems and other life experiences also play a part in pain. For example, women who have had babies are more pain-resistant than the rest of the population. An individual's ability to cope with challenges, emotional capability, and attitude toward physicians and medication can influence the perception of pain. Thoughts about not reaching your life goals due to the disease will also play a role in how you feel the pain. Conclusively, though emotions might not influence pain directly, they may increase awareness and vulnerability to discomfort. Again, social support from family and friends will go a long way to help alleviate a patient's pain.

Strategy for Pain Management

Nowadays, many pain management therapies can effectively reduce pain either alone or in combination. Caregivers will suggest specific treatments for specific sites or body parts. On the other hand, diffuse pain may require general treatment. One of the best ways to treat pain is to treat the underlying cause of the pain, which will eventually lead to limited or fewer side effects. This, therefore, reminds the patient to stay the course during their treatment plan from their doctor.

Some patients tend to withhold some information from their doctors or caregivers. It is advisable to always make sure the healthcare provider knows all the allergies you might be experiencing from medications. This will help avoid those medications that are not suitable for your system. Sometimes, if not properly handled, extreme allergies can result in death. Though your physician might have a preferred mode of treatment for your pain, the simplest and cheapest way to take medications is by mouth. For patients who are unable to swallow for one reason or the other, that is when another method should be considered. Try to avoid medications given intramuscularly because it hurts, is inconvenient, and absorption into your system might be unreliable.

Why Do You Have Pain

The pain a cancer patient might have might be because of either the cancer, the effects of the treatment, or a combination of the two. To give an effective treatment for the pain, it is important to understand the cause of the pain. It is not unusual throughout the treatment that the cause of the pain might change over time. Some cancer-related pain might be because of the growth and spread of the tumor. When cancer cells involve bones, muscles, nerves, or other organs, there is a likelihood that pain might occur.

Experiences have also shown that pain from cancer-related treatments is equally frequent. For instance, pain from surgery sometimes exists long after the surgery, though as the body heals, the pain diminishes. Pain from the effects of radiation after radiation therapy is equally very common. This is most noticeable in patients treated for breast and head and neck cancers. Some chemotherapy drugs also have side effects, which might lead to pain, like a burning sensation in the hands and feet.

It is noted as well that being confined to a bed might lead to complications like constipation and bed sores, which are uncomfortable. Moreover, emotions from bed confinement might lead to pain as well. In addition to cancer, some percentage of people might have other illnesses or disorders that produce pain, such as headaches or degenerative diseases. All these complications and other symptoms throughout the course of your treatment should be addressed promptly and accordingly.

Pain Relief

There is no definite approach toward pain relief. There is always constant reevaluation and if one approach is not working, your healthcare provider or doctor will move on to another approach. This is also always common sense to improve your symptoms. The patient should be practical and able to keep their approach as simple as possible. Complicated regimens, such as multiple medications that must be taken frequently at different times of the day, should be avoided. This leads to a patient carrying many medications around while continually watching the clock as if they are timekeepers.

Pain control should involve all hands on deck, and continuing care is very crucial to its success. The oncology staff should work hand in hand with the social worker, primary care doctor, and other caregivers in the team to provide consistent and aggressive pain relief in the hospital and or other settings convenient for the patient. In a nutshell, avoid confusion between multiple providers.

It is noted that in many instances, cancer therapy removes or shrinks the tumor and thus eliminates any pain that might originate from that part of the body. Palliative treatment is prescribed to alleviate pain, and radiation therapy happens to be one of the fastest and most effective methods of relieving pain, especially if the pain is caused by bone metastases. Other pain relief methods include surgery, such as tumor resection, drainage of abscesses, and treatment of bowel obstruction, which are helpful in relieving pain.

CHAPTER 5
Sexuality

Sexuality is an aspect of life that, in some cases, is the most uncomfortable topic to talk about, and changes that have taken place because of the cancer a patient has. Many patients report having less sex than before they had the disease. Nonetheless, according to experiences, pleasurable feelings and sexual performance can continue in some form or the other for almost everyone. Couples or partners may have to do things differently to increase or stimulate their better half. They may change positions or habits or adapt to new ways of expressing caring to meet each other's sexual or intimate needs. Cancer patients of both sexes must deal with their feelings about their bodies and the effect of these on their self-esteem. There should be open discussion on cancer as a disease, sexuality, and treatment among cancer patients and their partners because it is crucial and an integral part of life. Every individual's experience might be different. Thus, getting an accurate diagnosis of a patient's sexual problem is very important.

Effects of Cancer on Sexuality

To have good sexual intercourse or response involves a combination of factors that converge in the brain. The blood vessels, nerves, hormones, sex organs, and senses should all focus in that direction. It does not matter how attractive your partner might look; if one or more of the above is compromised, intercourse will not be as smooth. An individual should be able to clear their mind to have good-quality sex. For some people with cancer, it might be difficult to achieve orgasm, at least temporarily. Talking to two of my patients who were undergoing radiation therapy about sex, the male patient who was having his prostate treated told me he could have sex at any time, depending on the position he found his wife at that moment. The female patient, on the other hand, who was having her breast irradiated, said the last time she had sex was last night, but her husband had to work harder to bring her to the mood.

Physical Disorder

Cancer can disrupt sex if there is any physical disorder in the individual's body, either due to the disease itself or through the treatment process. It is not unusual for blood vessels, sex organs, glands, or nerves necessary for sex to be damaged in one way or the other. During surgical procedures, some blood vessels might be removed or destroyed, and organs and nerves distorted. Sometimes, during chemotherapy and radiation therapy, especially if the lower part of the body, like the pelvic area, is treated, blood flow around the genitals might be affected. Nerve function around this part of the body is usually affected, too. Hormone therapy may directly affect the chemical balance of the body necessary for a better sexual response. Many drugs taken during chemotherapy can cause vomiting. Nausea, fatigue, and even pain can interfere with sexuality. It is equally possible that some of the medications taken to counteract some of the side effects from the above complications can be detrimental to sexual arousal.

To try to overcome some or any inhibitions you might have during or after the course of your cancer treatment, bring up the sex topic when discussing with your physician. Bringing up sexual concerns will reduce surprises. Equally, discussing this with your nurse, doctor, or social worker might lead to some other resources that might be very helpful for your case. Remember, other patients have been or are going through your same route today.

Psychological and Emotional Concerns

Emotional and psychological disorders are some of the main causes of sexual problems for cancer patients. Due to medical advancements and research, if properly diagnosed, sexual anxieties can be treated. The last thing that will occur in the mind of a patient diagnosed with cancer is sex. This is because it is psychologically and emotionally depressing to the patient to the extent that a patient might feel they are no longer attractive to their partners. In most cases, cancer patients are depressed. The fact that an individual is depressed, their mind is taken off sex. There is, equally, the fear factor involved. The fact that a patient feels it might be very painful if they have sex, especially females who are having their pelvic area treated with radiation, the desire diminishes.

Sometimes, there is an alteration in the body image of the individual who has cancer. A woman who has lost a breast to cancer or has undergone facial changes might feel very unattractive. This eventually leads to low self-esteem and, consequently, loss of sexual desire. A man whose testicles have been tampered with might also lose desire for sex and, consequently, experience fewer erections. Talking to some of my patients about sex, women have less concern about sexual habits than men. African men, on the other hand, tend to be more concerned about their sexuality than the rest of the population. They want to preserve their sex organs even if it means compromising their treatment. Women who have lost their hair from treatment, especially chemotherapy, feel unattractive, and that is why most women on treatment will put on artificial hair and other forms of artificial parts for their breasts. The fact that a patient is undergoing treatment sometimes might equally affect their partners. A partner might feel it could be very painful to have sex with a cancer patient, or the fact that a body part might have been altered makes the partner unattractive. Divorces have taken place both during and immediately after cancer treatment. This is more prevalent among men than women. I have had patients tell me how their husbands have left them because they believe they can't make love to them, or they are no longer sexually attractive.

Professional Help

Unfortunately, most healthcare professionals, including doctors and nurses, are not comfortable discussing sexuality with their patients. On the other hand, I feel it is important for them to be more proactive in educating patients on issues regarding sex, especially if they must tamper with the patient's body image or sex organs. This will help the patient to learn how to manage their sex life. Many patients feel that doctors who, from experience, know the outcome or effect on the patient's sexuality should have sex discussions with their patients, especially those who are still sexually active.

Though the issue of sex might be too sensitive to discuss, it is the role of the healthcare facility that is providing treatment to a patient to recommend the help of sex therapists, psychologists, or psychiatrists who might help patients to open up. Opening a line of communication by initially discussing anything pertaining to the patient's treatment or extracurricular activities and, eventually, what to expect sexually, will go a long way in helping the patient and partner know what to expect.

The importance of support groups should not be underestimated. Remember, these are people either going through what you are right now or have had the same disease you now have. Thus, having discussions about other things, including sex, will help create intimacy and an exchange of experiences, which will be very helpful to you as a patient. A patient will be very surprised by the amount of useful information they will derive from this group, which will be very helpful in their bedroom or how to derive sexual pleasure.

Other Options

The effects of cancer treatment on sexuality can be very damaging to the patient. Exploring other ways to experience this desire or passion is just as valid as traditional intercourse involving the penis and vagina. The population that is engaging in oral sex is more than you might think. Oral sex is acceptable and can be substituted for traditional intercourse. Oral sex may allow tender parts of your body to heal while providing gratification to keep both partners happy. The downside of oral sex could be HPV, which can be contracted from this act. This could lead to having a form of head and neck cancer (ACS, 2019).

Another option could be masturbation. Masturbation is when an individual palpates their sex organs to achieve orgasm. Though both men and women will use this mode for satisfaction, it is easier for men than it is for women. Men can use their hands to palpate on their penis with a high concentration of imagination, and before you know it, they are ejaculating. Women, on the other hand, will need a very comfortable spot to either sit or lie down and might need an object to use in the process. Many of my patients have used this form of sexual arousal, especially single females. They are very comfortable with it and, in most cases, don't have to look for outside partners or men. ("I don't need a man," they will say.) Again, masturbation is a legitimate mode of sexual activity to release and comfort as well.

Sex Therapist

A sex therapist is a trained professional with a mental health and sexuality certification. This professional will study your situation and will be able to work with you to help solve your problem. A sex therapist does not mean this individual will be or will want to have sex with you. He or she is like any healthcare professional you will meet throughout your cancer treatment journey.

Questions for Your Doctor

- How will this treatment affect my sexuality or ability to perform?

- Will I be able to have children after my treatment?

- What other options do I have for my sexuality or the ability to have children?

- As a woman, will this lead to early menopause?

- Be sure to discuss the benefits and risks associated with the medication, device, or implant you might have to help in your sexual activity.

CHAPTER 6
Cancer Prevention

Scientists are very active in research to prevent cancer before it happens, especially if there are risk factors like genetics in the family or when a carcinogenic process has started. Chemical trials are also underway to determine the effectiveness of certain chemo preventions, that is, the process of using certain preventive agents to stop the growth of some indicative cancer cells. They are looking for a possibility to suppress cancer by inhibiting the proliferation of abnormal cells. Research also shows that scientists are beginning to identify some of the mutations that set the stage for cancer development. This is noticeable in the hereditary form of breast and colon cancers. Scientists are therefore building on this knowledge to help reverse and or halt cancer genes from developing. Preventing cancer completely is highly unachievable, but certain cancers can be prevented, at least to a greater extent (ACS, 2019).

Breast Cancer

The chances of having breast cancer can be prevented or minimized, if not by more than half of the studies if certain guidelines are followed. Regardless of whether you have a history of breast cancer in the family or not, especially for women who are of childbearing age and above, the following will be helpful (NCI, 2019).

Firstly, practice breast self-examination. Breast self-examination is a situation whereby an individual palpates their breast to feel if there is any abnormality, such as a node or lump. This should be done once a month by raising one hand and using the other or the opposite hand to palpate the opposite breast. This should be done regularly, and any abnormality should be reported to your primary care physician.

Secondly, the frequency of mammographic screening is based on guidelines by the American Cancer Society. Mammography is the X-ray of the breast. Occasionally, there are controversies about whether mammograms are very helpful in preventing breast cancer. Of course, the advantage of having an annual mammogram, especially for women of childbearing age, outweighs the disadvantages, if there are any. Usually, if any abnormality, such as nodules, is detected on the mammographic X-ray, a further evaluation, such as a biopsy, is recommended (ACS, 2019).

The consumption of a lower-fat and well-balanced diet can be very helpful in preventing breast cancer. Exercising regularly and preventing being overweight will be helpful not only in cancer prevention but also in overall health. If, for some reason, there is any abnormal discharge from your breast, take it very seriously. Again, if there is any abnormality on your breast, do not hesitate to talk to your doctor or seek a second opinion. A colleague of mine was diagnosed with breast cancer thanks to her persistence in seeking answers about an abnormality in her breast, even after consulting multiple doctors.

Colorectal Cancer

Colorectal cancer is cancer of the large intestine (colon) and the rectum. The combination of the name is because the rectum is the last portion of the large intestine. Although colorectal cancer is the third highest type of cancer affecting people in the United States, the number of deaths is decreasing. Over the years, the rate of recurrences has equally decreased. This is partly due to preventive measures and advancements in screening methods (ACS, 2019).

Fecal Occult Blood Test

Colorectal cancer is associated with polyps, a growth in the large intestine or colon that leads to bleeding. To rule out colon cancer, bleeding, or the breakdown products in the feces are tested. Several types of tests are available for detecting fecal occult blood. All these techniques are geared toward identifying hemoglobin, a component in the blood.

The guaiac-based fecal occult blood test uses the chemical guaiac to detect blood in the stool. This test, which is done once a year, is a situation in which an individual receives a take-home kit from a healthcare provider. A brush or stick is used to obtain a small amount of stool. This is subsequently returned to the lab or the hospital, where the sample is tested for blood in the stool. The Fecal Immunochemical test, which uses antibodies to detect blood in the stool, is another type of stool test. Another method of testing blood in the stool is the FIT-DNA Test. This detects if there is any alteration of DNA in the stool. This is a test whereby you collect the whole bowel movement and send it to the lab, where it is checked for cancer cells. Its interval is between one and three years.

Sigmoidoscopy

Sigmoidoscopy is a procedure in which a flexible, narrow tube called an endoscope is gently inserted into the rectum and passed upwards into the sigmoid colon to detect growth. If any growths or polyps are detected, they can be removed using the same instrument.

Colonoscopy

This is a situation whereby an examination of your colon is performed, like the sigmoidoscopy above, but this goes further. In a colonoscopy, X-rays of the colon are taken using the inserted tube through your rectum and displayed on the computer to detect polyps. Usually, a day before this exam, an individual is advised to empty the bowels by using Fleet or laxatives and usually go with an empty stomach for a day as preparation for the procedure, except for drinking fluids.

Questions for Your Doctor

If you are at risk, talk to your doctor.

- What test is right for me?
- When do I begin testing?
- How often should I get tested?
- What is the worst outcome of having a colonoscopy?
- Is it possible to know how long the anesthesiologist has practiced?
- What are the qualifications of the anesthesiologist?
- Do people usually have any reaction from having a colonoscopy?

Diet and Nutrition

The importance of eating a healthy diet cannot be underestimated when it comes to preventing colorectal cancer. Eating high-fiber, low-fat meals reduces the risk of colorectal cancer. Avoid as much fat as possible from meat and animals. Good nutritional habits are also a good preventive measure for other forms of cancer (ACS, 2019).

It is recommended that screening for colorectal cancer should begin at age 50, or if you are at risk, especially if you have a family history of the disease, much earlier. Making screening decisions is the best part of cancer detection. It is, therefore, important to get counseling services, screening, and preventive medicine as much as possible.

Cervical Cancer

Cervical cancer is one of those gynecological cancers that is preventable or at least the risk minimized. In most cervical cancer cases, an individual has already contracted the disease before seeing the symptoms. Early screening habits and methods help prevent or reduce the risk of having this form of cancer.

Pap smear

A pap smear is the examination of abnormal cells under the microscope that are removed from a woman's cervix. This is normal for women of childbearing age in a healthcare environment.

To get the specimen, the vagina is spread open by a paddle or speculum, and a cotton swab or tiny spatula sweeps across the cervix to remove some cells. This specimen is then smeared on a glass slide, dipped into a preservative, and sent to a laboratory for testing. Usually, a cytotechnologist examines this under a microscope, but recently, the analysis has been done by computer due to the advancement in technology. To ensure accuracy, intercourse should be avoided 24 hours before the procedure. It is also recommended that douching and any medications, including vaginal contraceptives, should be avoided at least three days before the examination. To avoid false negative results, testing should be done in a reputable lab. On the other hand, since it takes about three years for normal cells to become cancerous, it is possible that if false negative results occur, they will be caught in subsequent years. The American Cancer Society recommends that a woman of childbearing age start having their pap smear done either if they begin sexual activities or at the age of 18, whichever comes first.

Endometrial Tissue Sample

Endometrial cancer, according to scientists, is on the rise; as a matter of fact, it is one of the most common types of female genital cancer. A biopsy or sample of endometrial tissue is removed from the endometrium, the lining of the uterus, through a tube or suction tube or a spoon-like instrument called a curette. There is no preparation for this examination, though a painkiller may be necessary. The American Cancer Society recommends endometrial tissue sampling for women at high risk of menopause. This includes women who are obese, have a history of infertility, abnormal uterine bleeding, and failure to ovulate on tamoxifen and estrogen therapies. Again, though this exam is mostly for a category of high-risk older women, other females can equally have this test, but at menopause.

Custom, Sex, and Reproductive Behaviors

Backgrounds and choices are sometimes risk factors for the cause of cervical cancer. This might affect the individuals personally, their families, or their children. For example, male children who are circumcised reduce the risk of having cancer for themselves and their future partners. The female partners of circumcised males have a lower risk of cervical cancer than those whose partners are uncircumcised. This could be due to HPV or poor hygiene. Promiscuity, which is the behavior of having multiple sex partners, exposes a female to sexually transmitted diseases like HPV, which eventually may lead to or increase the risk of cervical cancer (Murphy, G.P., Morris, L.B., & Lange, D., 1997).

Skin Cancer

Skin cancer is one of those cancers that we get mostly when we are having fun. That is when we are relaxing or feeling happy under the sunlight. Ultraviolet radiation from sunlight is one of the main causes of skin cancer. According to the American Cancer Society, skin cancer is becoming one of the most common types of cancer in the United States. More new cases of skin cancer are being diagnosed annually in the U.S.A. Most of the skin damage associated with aging, such as wrinkles, sagging, leathering, and discoloration, is ultraviolet-related. The damage from the sun is cumulative. That is why some of the tips listed below will either help reduce the risk or prevent it.

Clothing is one of the most effective defenses for protection. When you are going out there in the sun, especially in the afternoon or midday, wear densely woven and bright or dark-colored fabric. The more skin you cover, the better. So, choose long sleeves and pants whenever possible.

Tanning, either in the sun or in a salon, is never safe. Vitamin D is necessary for our health, but it is possible to obtain this vitamin from other sources, such as salmon, fortified milk, orange juice, and dietary supplements.

Wraparound sunglasses that block most of the sun's ultraviolet rays effectively shield both eyes and the surrounding skin. This helps prevent serious skin conditions, from cataracts to melanomas of the eye and eyelid. Hats with large brims equally offer significant protection for the face and back of the neck.

Sunscreen is also an important part of sun protection. It is advisable to look for a product that provides a sun-protective factor of 30 or higher. Use sunscreen whenever you are going outside in the sun, especially in all areas exposed to the sun. It is important to do skin self-evaluation to detect skin cancer early when it is most treatable. Seek medical advice on noticing susceptible spots on your skin. This equally applies to changes in the color of the skin, itching, or bleeding.

Babies or infants are susceptible to the sun's damaging effects because they possess little melanin, a pigment that gives color to skin, hair, and eyes and provides some sun protection. It is also advisable to provide babies with long sleeves or proper clothing when taking them outside. Covered umbrellas for strollers with hoods are equally recommended. Some protective sunscreens will be helpful for your baby.

CHAPTER 7
Cancer Prevention Among Youths

Humans go through many physical and social changes as they grow. These changes create opportunities for cancer prevention, especially those types of cancers that are hereditary. By addressing certain exposures and behaviors among the younger population today, we will be able to reduce the chances of cancer in the future. This can be accomplished based on the decisions and activities while young (ACS, 2019).

Radiation in Medicine

Medical imaging has become a big tool in medicine today. Physicians often use imaging procedures to determine the best option for treatment. Imaging procedures are medical tests that allow the doctor to see inside the body to diagnose, treat, and maintain a patient's health conditions. In the process, some of these procedures involve ionizing radiation, which can, in the future, present health risks to the patient. However, if patients understand the benefits and disadvantages of the procedure, they will be able to make an objective decision in choosing one particular type of medical imaging over the other.

Most people have had one form of medical imaging or another that produces or involves radiation. The type of procedure chosen by your physician will be based on your condition and the part of the body to be imaged. Some common imaging tests include computed tomography or CT scans and regular X-rays, including those at the dental clinic. Fluoroscopy, which is one of the highest militants of ionizing radiation, is losing steam due to more advanced technology. For your doctor to recommend one or any of the above imaging procedures, they should consider your age, the benefits, and the necessity of the procedure.

One of the conventional treatment types of cancer treatment today is the use of radiation therapy. Though radiation therapy is good for either cure or palliative treatment, it can also be a risk factor for cancer development in other parts of the body later in life.

Underage Drinking (Alcohol)

Alcohol is one of the most used and abused drugs among youths in the United States. Studies show that excessive drinking is responsible for at least 4,300 deaths among youths each year. (ACS, 2019). Though the legal age for the purchase of alcohol is 21, on average, youths drink more alcohol than adults on every drinking occasion. Although there is some evidence that alcohol is a carcinogen, it is sometimes a co-carcinogen because it seems to make other risk factors like tobacco use more harmful. Drinking heavily might lead to cirrhosis, which causes liver cancer. Studies, though still under research, show that there is equally a link between alcohol and breast cancer. From experience, alcohol consumption leads to unwanted, unplanned, and unprotected sexual activities, which increases the chances of HIV and HPV. Limiting alcohol use at a younger age is equally helpful in reducing the risk of contracting so many diseases, including cancer, later in life.

Tobacco

Tobacco use, which is associated with lung cancer, occurs more in heavy smokers than in the nonsmoking population. Cigarette use among the youth is increasing daily because it is a style or fashion among their peers. Tobacco, apart from causing lung cancer, can cause mouth, pharynx, larynx, esophagus, bladder, kidney, and pancreatic cancers (ACS, 2019). The many chemicals contained in cigarettes also enter the bloodstream, circulating to distant organs, thus affecting the bladder, kidney, and other organs. Having a discussion with your children on the consequences of these behaviors, which do not have any meaning in life, will go a long way in reducing the risk of this disease. Scientists are also discovering that secondhand smoke equally increases the risk of having cancer. Secondhand smoke is very prevalent in areas where people use cigars at nightclubs and bars. Avoid smoking at all costs to maintain good and quality health and avoid wasting money.

Diet

The lifestyle factor that has received the highest attention recently is diet. According to the American Cancer Society, it is suggested that about one-third of cancer deaths in the United States are associated with the diet factor. These include the type of food, portion sizes, preparatory methods, food variety, and caloric intake. High-fat diets and processed foods are associated with the risk of contracting cancer. Eating a diet rich in fruits and vegetables will be very helpful. Obesity, which typically is a consequence of eating too much fat and less sporting activity, also increases the risk of several cancers. Watching or maintaining a healthy weight balance or physical activities will help enhance a proper diet in reducing the disease. Again, eating fatty foods like fries and cakes should be avoided. When it comes to fried food like potatoes, it is not the potato component of the fries that is problematic but the cooking method. These foods are, in most cases, cooked in hydrogenated oils and are loaded with salt thereafter. In addition to salt and trans fats being a problem for your health, the high temperatures used to cook these foods result in high acrylamide levels (Informed Decisions, Murphy, G.P., Morris, L.B., & Lange, D., 1997). Acrylamide, a chemical present in industrial buildings and cigarette smoke, increases the risk of cancer. Again, moderate or good eating habits will be very helpful.

Fiber found in fruits, vegetables, and whole grains plays a key role in keeping your digestive system clean and healthy. It helps keep cancer-causing compounds moving through your digestive system or tract before they can cause great harm. Research has shown that eating a diet high in fiber may help prevent certain types of cancers, such as colorectal, stomach, and mouth cancers.

It is recommended that if you have a history of cancer in your family, making small changes to your diet and behaviors can make a big difference to your long-term health.

Preventive Surgery

Though it is not common, people inherit gene mutations that put them at risk of contracting cancer at an early age. Taking preventive measures to avoid this from happening is the way forward. In such cases, some people and their physicians may decide to take away an organ. I have seen cases whereby certain patients, including a co-worker, have taken off both their breasts to prevent breast cancer. This preventive measure is not common. It can sometimes be depressing in the long run to lose your body parts. My co-worker's husband did not take this lightly after the wife took away her breasts. Again, health comes first, as many people will say.

Environment

Various things can contribute to cancer if exposed to them often. Although major air pollutants do not show a strong link to cancer, asbestos is a well-established carcinogen. Some studies suggest that chlorination of water may have a link to the cause of cancer. Probably the most danger from pollution comes from the dangerous chemicals used in industries that escape into the surrounding environment. It is estimated that about one percent of cancers are linked to air, water, and land pollution. Not all these carcinogens affect everybody who is around lots of smoke or in a polluted environment will have, for example, lung cancer.

An unknown number of homes and office buildings contain invisible radioactive gas, which is associated with lung cancer. Sunlight or ultraviolet radiation poses a danger of skin cancer, especially to people with light skin. This hazard increases with altitude.

Vaccination

Cancer prevention also includes protection from certain viral infections. It is usually important to talk to your primary care physician about some of these.

Hepatitis B can increase the risk of developing liver cancer. The Hepatitis B vaccine is recommended for certain individuals who might be at high risk. This includes people who are sexually active and might have more than one partner. The rate of people having more than one sexual partner could be high among youths, which might be very dangerous if they are exposed to sexually transmitted diseases. People who use intravenous drugs, men who sleep with men, and healthcare workers who could be exposed to Hepatitis B should equally be vaccinated.

HPV is a sexually transmitted virus that can lead to cervical and other genital cancers, as well as some head and neck cancers. HPV vaccines are recommended for boys and girls between the ages of 11 and 12. On the other hand, it is not too late to take these vaccines if you think you are at high risk (ACS, 2019).

Avoid Risky Behaviors

Other effective ways of cancer prevention include avoiding risky behaviors that can lead to infections, which might eventually lead to cancer.

The practice of safe sex by limiting the number of sexual partners and ensuring the use of condoms during intercourse is undoubtedly a good practice. The more sexual partners you have in your lifetime, the more likely you are to contract a sexually transmitted disease such as HPV and human immunodeficiency virus (HIV). Research has shown that people who have HIV have a higher risk of having lung, liver, and anal cancers. HPV is often associated with the penis, head and neck, and some other gynecological cancers (ACS, 2019).

The practice of avoiding sharing needles cannot be underestimated in its importance. Sharing needles with people who use intravenous drugs can lead to HIV as well as Hepatitis B, which can increase the risk of liver cancer. There is professional attention available to those who are concerned or addicted to drug use.

Maintain a Healthy Weight

Obesity makes an individual not only physically unfit but also unhealthy. Maintaining a healthy weight might lower the risk of contracting some types of cancers, including kidney, breast, lung, prostate, and colorectal cancers. Many physical activities also help to reduce the risk of colon and breast cancers (ACS 2019). Strive to do some moderate and vigorous aerobic activities every week. Also, make a goal to include thirty or more minutes of physical activity in your daily routine.

Hereditary Awareness

A family history of cancer is one of the best predictors of the disease. However, according to studies, primary preventive efforts are often undermined or not targeted to individuals who have the greatest risk. The lack of or inadequate targeted primary prevention behavioral interventions reflects the reality that all individuals are susceptible to cancer regardless of having a history or not.

The question now is which is the best way to deliver these cancer-preventive messages to those at a high risk based on family history. Cardiovascular diseases, as well as some other diseases, have used family-based interventions to prevent these diseases from being passed to family members. Targeting family members for cancer prevention may be a useful strategy as family members may be more motivated, capitalizing as teachable tools to those at higher risk in the same environment or gene or both. We believe that the potential is greater to increase cancer prevention efforts by starting earlier in life in the family to complement other community preventive efforts. Again, this home-based pattern, if well implemented, will be handed down from one generation to another. In a nutshell, it becomes a family recipe.

General Rule of Thumb

As a youth, regular self-exams and screening for various types of cancers such as skin, colon, breast, and cervix can increase your chances of discovering cancer early enough when it is still localized and curable. It is advisable to always find out from your doctor the types of cancers you should be screened for at every stage of your life.

Questions to your Doctor

- How much radiation am I getting from dental or other medical X-rays?

- Can I have a shield whenever I am having X-rays?

- What types of cancers can I prevent at my age?

- Do I have a history of any cancer in my family?

- What are some of the dangerous behaviors I can avoid to prevent cancer at my age?

- How can I find out if there is a history of cancer in my family?

CHAPTER 8
Signs and Symptoms of Cancer

Like so many other diseases, cancer is progressive in nature. Some symptoms occur earlier when a tumor is growing in a structure or an organ, and as the cancer grows, it produces new signs and symptoms involving new organs. It is not unusual for other symptoms to arise from the immune system fighting to get rid of the malignant cells.

Having one sign or symptom does not necessarily mean someone has one disease or the other. This information may not be enough to draw one conclusion or another. However, if an individual has multiple symptoms and signs, such as blood in the urine and frequent urination, which is not because of frequent drinking, then a physician may get a better picture of what is going on. It could be your bladder, uterus, prostate, etc. Sometimes, even with additional symptoms and signs, the doctor might not get a clear picture of what is happening. That is why they may recommend X-rays, blood tests, and biopsy or refer a patient to other specialists for further evaluation.

How Does Cancer Cause Signs and Symptoms?

There is no one path, but cancer is noted to be a group of diseases that can cause almost any sign or symptom. Usually, the signs and symptoms will depend on where the cancer is, its size, and how it affects the organs or tissues. Sometimes, signs and symptoms may appear in different parts of the body. This, therefore, means that the cancer has spread. It is not unusual for cancer to spread to other parts of the body before the initial diagnosis. As cancer grows, it spreads to other organs, surrounding tissues, nerves, and blood vessels. The pressure from this push might be a symptom or sign of cancer. Some parts of the body are very sensitive, like the eyes and brain, and even the smallest tumor might be a sign or symptom of the disease (ACS, 2019).

Certain cancers do not cause any signs or symptoms until they have grown too large. In most cases, such cancers are not curable. Examples of such cancers are the spleen and pancreatic cancers. In the case of pancreatic cancer, which happens to be one of the deadliest forms of cancer, the signs, which include back and belly pain, come in when it is late. Jaundice, which is caused by the growth around the bile, leads to the blockage of the bile duct, thus reducing bile flow, causing yellow eyes and skin as signs.

Weight loss, fever, fatigue, and extreme tiredness are some symptoms caused by cancer. This may be because cancer cells use or eat up most of the body's energy supply. It can also be due to the release of a substance that changes the way the body makes energy from food. It is also possible that the immune system is affected, and one will experience these signs and symptoms, too.

Studies have also shown that sometimes cancer cells release substances into the bloodstream that are not usually linked to the cancer. It is noted that some cancers of the pancreas do release substances that cause blood clots in the veins of the legs. Sometimes, people's nerves and muscles are affected, and they feel weak and dizzy. This is because of some hormone-like substances that raise the blood calcium caused by some form of lung cancer (ACS, 2019).

Some Signs and Symptoms Footnotes

The likelihood of treating and curing cancer when it is still localized, that is, when it has not yet spread to other parts of the body, is very high. At this point, the removal of this spot through surgery might be the only mode of treatment required. That is why it is necessary to see the doctor immediately after starting to experience some of those signs and symptoms.

Breast cancer happens to be one of those cancers that can easily be treated. Immediately, if you feel a lump or cyst in your breast, don't think it will go away on its own. Contact your physician as soon as possible. Skin cancer is another form of cancer that can easily be treated before it spreads to other parts of the body. Consult your doctor immediately if you see an unusual spot on your skin.

People tend to ignore some of these signs and symptoms. Though those symptoms might not mean anything, they shouldn't be ignored. The outcome of wasting time might haunt you for the rest of your life. Never be frustrated about the outcome if you check into a hospital. It will not be worse than if it turns out to be cancer in the future. Money may be a determining factor in why people will not seek medical attention. Take yourself to an emergency room. It is also true that some signs and symptoms that are cancer signs, like weakness, tiredness, and coughing, might not be cancer-related. But if, for one reason or the other, they are long-term and are not going away, they may be a cancer concern sign.

The American Cancer Society recommends that people should visit their doctors for cancer-related checkups. This is because it is possible to find cancer before the manifestation of any signs or symptoms. Mammograms are recommended for women 40 years and above for breast cancer screening. Pelvic exams and pap smears are recommended for sexually active women for gynecological cancer screening. Colon cancer screening, like colonoscopy, is also recommended for people 45 years and above, especially if you have a history of colon cancer in your family.

Some Other Signs and Symptoms

Cancer signs and symptoms are mostly common signs we experience daily. This does not mean that they might not be something else. If they persist, especially in a combination over a long period of time, visit or consult a doctor.

Fever

Continuous fever has been associated with cancer. This is because the immune system has been compromised either by the disease or treatment. It is noted that people with Hodgkin's disease usually have an elevated temperature most of the time (ACS, 2019). These patients' temperature fluctuates between higher than normal and returning to normal. The fact that the immune system is compromised makes it difficult to fight the cancer. It is also noted, though to a lesser extent, that fever may also be a sign of other cancers like leukemia and liver cancer. High fever sometimes occurs in the presence of secondary cancers like lung, kidney, pancreas, and cancer of the gastrointestinal tract (ACS, 2019).

Fever is also an indication of secondary infection and, if very high, can cause sweating, malaise, and sometimes even confusion. Sometimes, fever also indicates that the body or the immune system is fighting an infection.

Unexplained Weight Loss

Sometimes, unexplained weight loss may be a sign of cancer. It is noted that a loss of 10 pounds or above in a month may be a sign of cancer. Cancers of the pancreas, esophagus, kidney, and lung are the cancers most associated with a lot of weight loss (Murphy, G.P., Morris, L.B., & Lange, D., 1997).

It has been noted that a couple of aspects of cancer lead to weight loss. Tumors sometimes directly affect the functioning of the digestive system by preventing the body from absorbing the entire nutrient from the foods we eat. It is also noted that some tumors expand rapidly and appear to grow independently of the host and draw nutrients from healthy tissues.

As tumors grow, they trigger an increase in the burning of calories. As they divide, they require a lot of energy, and the metabolic process is equally accelerated, which also leads to the loss of excessive energy. It is also noted that since people with cancer don't always have the appetite to eat, either due to the disease itself or treatment, the supply of energy cannot meet the demands of the body (ACS, 2019).

Pain

Pain is noted to be a sign or symptom of cancer. In some cases, it is because of the tumor's destruction of healthy tissues, the obstruction of an organ, pressure, infection, or the stretching of internal organs and structures. Pain is sometimes noted to be the beginning signs of cancers like bladder, which makes urination painful, and lung, whereby a patient experiences pain in the arm, shoulder, upper back, and chest. Tumors of the eye, brain, and or the sinuses may also cause pain by pressing on the nerves and blood vessels.

Sometimes, the location of pain associated with cancer does not always reveal the actual location of the tumor. This is because the body is linked with a network of nerves that feed into a central interpretation system by the brain. Pain from one part of the body may be coming from another part. For example, pain from stomach cancer might be felt in the chest.

Fatigue

Extreme tiredness that does not get better even after rest is known as fatigue. This is sometimes caused by weight loss. Fatigue is not a significant symptom or sign of cancer except when the cancer is advanced. Another cause of fatigue might be extreme blood loss, which may not be associated with cancer, though colon and stomach cancers are often connected to this symptom. It is also noted that fatigue becomes more symptomatic with the growth or advancement of cancer.

Skin Signs

Sometimes, cancer can cause visible signs and symptoms on the human skin. Skin cancer starts as a mole or growth that doesn't heal. An example of such a malignancy is melanoma. Such growth tends to spread to every direction of the body while equally changing colors.

Studies have shown that, though to a lesser extent, a growth on the skin can be a metastasis resulting from another cancer such as lung, breast, stomach, kidney, and ovaries. (ACS, 2019). Some of the characteristics of such modules are either reddish or bluish in color and are mostly located near the site of the primary cancers. Other signs on the skin include patchy hair loss and darkening of the skin, especially under the arms or lower back, neck, and groin. Darkening of the skin is linked to cancers of the gastrointestinal tract, prostate, uterus, kidney, and ovary. Lymphomas, leukemia, cervical, breast, and lung cancers are also linked to erythema or skin reddening (Murphy, G.P., Morris, L.B., & Lange, D., 1997).

Persistent itching is also among the common signs of cancer. Continued or prolonged itching that doesn't go away may be a sign of Hodgkin's disease, as well as carcinomas of the pancreas, brain, stomach, adrenal gland, or ovary (ACS, 2019).

Some Other Signs and Symptoms

Some other common signs and symptoms should also be watched for, for they might suggest cancer. This might be a direct result of either a primary or a metastatic cancer. They may occur because cancer causes the overproduction of hormones or when the tumor produces and or secretes substances. This process, called toxohormones, may have effects on some body organs like the spleen and liver. Fever might come up because of the release of a pyrogenic substance from the tumor. Hyperpigmentation is noted to be due to the excess production of melanocyte-stimulating hormones (Murphy, G.P., Morris, L.B., & Lange, D., 1997).

Studies also show that there is a possibility of cancer tumors releasing toxic substances that affect the neurologic and muscular systems. A situation called carcinomatous neuromyopathy usually affects some patients who have lung, cervical, breast, ovarian, prostate, and colon cancers. Muscle weakness and wasting are the most common manifestations of carcinomatous neuromyopathy (Murphy, G.P., Morris, L.B., & Lange, D., 1997). Again, it is important to talk to your doctor whenever you see or experience any of these signs or symptoms over a long period of time.

Changes in your Mood

Anxiety and depression can be produced by physical illness that can come about by influencing hormones and brain chemicals. Pancreatic cancers are noted to be some of those cancers that can produce the above symptoms. It is not unusual for symptoms like depression, anxiety, and insomnia to appear before any physical symptoms or signs. Pancreatic cancer does not produce any early signs until it is well advanced. A series of mood changes can be an indication of this disease (ACS, 2019).

The population is being advised to pay attention to anxiety, depression, and other emotional signs and symptoms that might appear from nowhere. But also be advised that when these signs persist, see the doctor.

Alarming Signs and Symptoms

There are some alarming signs or symptoms that one shouldn't overlook for a long time. Though they might be false positive signs, do not wait. Take yourself to the doctor immediately and get checked. These signs are noted to be important cancer warnings. Most developed countries' cancer organizations, including the American Cancer Society, have established a couple of common clues to watch.

Unusual Bleeding and Discharge

Unusual bleeding is not a good sign, and it is noted to occur at any stage of cancer development. It can occur either at an early or advanced stage of the disease. Vaginal bleeding periods at any time after menopause should be of great concern. Any woman who experiences excessive bleeding at any time, especially during periods, should see their doctor immediately. These may be cancer warning signs. Cancers of the uterus and cervix can cause vaginal bleeding. A bloody discharge from the nipple may indicate breast cancer. Blood in the urine may be a sign of either bladder or kidney cancer. Colon and rectal cancers are manifested by blood in the stool. Blood in one's cough could be a signal for lung cancer.

Thickening or Lump on the Body

The development of a tumor can be felt through the skin. This is mostly noticed on the breast, soft tissues of the body, or testicles. Self-body examination or palpation of your body parts, like the axillaries, breasts, and testicles, is recommended by the American Cancer Society. It is possible that you have detected a tumor at an earlier stage if you report any unusual thickening or lump to your doctor before it spreads to other parts of the body.

Unusual Sores

Sometimes, cancers, especially those of the skin, may bleed and resemble sores that never heal. Sores may come up anywhere on the body, but mostly in the mouth and the genitals. It is necessary or important to have them evaluated immediately when they are noticed. Sometimes, these sores become malignant, especially if one is involved in any cancer-causing activities such as chewing or smoking tobacco and heavy alcohol intake.

Nagging Cough or Hoarseness

Nagging cough and persistent hoarseness may suggest cancer of the lung or thyroid. If you are experiencing this condition, contact your physician. If you cough persistently for two weeks or more, it might be a sign of cancer.

Recent Changes in a Wart or Mole

Most people are usually in a state of denial. It is recommended that any wart or mole on your body that changes color, size, or shape be reported to the doctor as soon as possible. A skin change may be a sign of cancer, which, if detected early enough, can be cured. On the other hand, it might not be cancer-related, but the rule of thumb is that it should be reported.

Indigestion or Swallowing Difficulties

Usually, in situations with signs of indigestion and difficulties swallowing, it might indicate the presence of cancer. Cancers of the stomach, esophagus, or pharynx are sometimes associated with these signs (ACS, 2019). Again, it may not be cancer-related, but it is necessary to contact a doctor if you experience these signs over a long period of time.

Footnotes

Most people are often in a state of denial whenever they experience signs and symptoms of lung cancer. They might attribute it to changes in eating habits or stress due to a heavy workload. In a nutshell, people deny the fact that something is wrong, and they even postpone doctor's appointments and checkups. See a doctor, and don't be in denial. I would prefer to be told it is nothing to be concerned about than being diagnosed with stage 4 cancer.

Timing is crucial in cancer care. Human beings tend to believe that symptoms will disappear. It is not until the symptoms interfere with their daily life activities, like too much pain, that they act. Be proactive about your health. The rule of thumb on cancer is that if it is not prevented, the earlier it is caught or diagnosed, the better for the patient.

It is not unusual for some people to be frightened by the loss of independence that goes with a disease like cancer. They are not comfortable with the weakness that might result from chemotherapy or radiation therapy treatment. Being helpless and or dependent on family, friends, and doctors may be other fears. Hair loss, losing one or more breasts from breast cancer, and even a lack of sexual desire might be a concern to some patients, especially females. I have had patients of both sexes whose spouses have divorced them because they have breast and prostate cancer, respectively. Sometimes, rather than denial, people respond with anger, guilt, and or depression. Bear in mind that you are not alone or the first person in your situation, and reacting quickly to your situation is the best thing to do.

CHAPTER 9
The Cancer Team Approach

When someone is diagnosed with cancer, they automatically believe they have come to the end of their life. This might be due to the complexity of what it takes or the stages and steps involved.

From diagnosis to treatment to recovery, cancer care involves a continuum of healthcare professionals who provide various skills in the cancer treatment and recovery journey. The location where the care can be offered varies. This includes doctors' offices to hospitals, from specialized hospitals to your residence or home. Due to the level of technology and the large number of people involved, it is important that there should be a coordinator or communication to meet your medical, emotional, and practical needs and those of your family. One of my former patients who was undergoing both external radiation therapy and chemotherapy was about to have brachytherapy in another hospital for her cervical cancer without notifying either physician. This could have been a double exposure or treatment with lots of unrevised damages, which could lead to death.

Previously, cancer management had been a straightforward process. Perhaps your doctor could detect your disease during your routine visit and refer you to a cancer specialist. But nowadays, the situation has changed due to the advances in treatment, with the development of the oncology specialty and considering the vast need of patient and family health concerns as only part of the picture. This is because people with cancer need help with psychological, social, financial, and occupational concerns as well. From diagnosis through recovery requires far more expertise than any single caregiver can provide. Thus, many professionals and even cancer survivors serve as volunteers as soon as they are diagnosed.

Your Care Coordinator

Cancer care is overwhelming; thus, most patients would like to have a coordinator to coordinate their treatment. The coordinator will act as a liaison throughout the process and will evaluate the development. The process has become so complex due to the number of steps and the many professionals involved. To manage your illness, you will need to identify a coordinator to help you throughout the course of your treatment.

Your primary care doctor will be a priority of choice as a coordinator to most patients. Your primary care physician knows you very well, and probably it is this doctor who discovered your disease or their setting and is in a better place to recommend you to an oncologist or group they are familiar with and confident he or she will be able to handle your type of cancer. Secondly, your primary care physician is the doctor who will be taking care of or seeing you both during and after treatment and will be able to monitor your progress.

From experience, most primary care doctors will accept the responsibility or role of their patient's coordinator. On the other hand, not every patient has a personal doctor. It is possible that some patients were diagnosed with the disease after checking in an emergency room. In the absence of a primary care doctor, the oncologist whom you were referred to might accept to carry on this role.

You can select your spouse, partner, friend, etc. This individual can accompany you to all your appointments if possible. This companion should be able to ask questions on your behalf, remember information, or write down instructions. Your coordinator might become the center of your support group, coordinating among friends and family. It is, therefore, imperative to choose an individual who will be available long-term and have a good knowledge of your medical history. It will also be advantageous if your coordinator has an idea of medical terminology and who, for example, might understand what cure and palliative treatment mean.

The Patient's Participation

The patient's total participation and involvement are very crucial. For the team to provide the best of care throughout your treatment and recovery journey, you should keep in mind that you are the team captain and not the coach or the coordinator. The role of the coordinator should be that of the physician, preferably your primary care doctor.

Bear in mind that as part of your team, you will decide which procedure or treatment offers you the best care and the highest quality of life. But you will only decide what is good for you after others have provided information, alternatives, and recommendations. Your acceptance or refusal is final, but on the other hand, it is not unusual to delegate some of these responsibilities of decision-making to a trusted family member or sometimes a longtime friend to make such decisions on your behalf.

As you progress in the decision-making process, there will be alternative opinions; listen to them all before making a decision. Moreover, not all that you will be told will be what you would like to hear. Know very well that you will be dealing with a lot of professionals with many experiences, of which your case is one of the many cases they have seen, and yours has been one of the least bad cases they have seen. Always bear in mind that you are sick, want to be cured, and that the people working for you are there to serve your interests. They may not conduct business your way or the way you want but never frustrate them. I have had patients who thought I didn't know what I was doing but later became my best friends. Saying "Sorry for my behavior the other day" to a healthcare worker taking care of you doesn't hurt.

Some patients also tend to take control of their care and learn every detail of their disease. This is done by internet research or talking to other people, like survivors and other specialists until it fits their situation. There is also this group of people who will rely on the advice of experts to whom they have entrusted major decisions and care. They may feel ill-equipped to comprehend and absorb every detail and are satisfied for others to analyze and evaluate the technicalities and present them with recommendations.

Again, no matter what role you are comfortable with, always have the right mindset, express yourself, and obtain the information you require for informed decisions. Your world is not over, a feeling most cancer patients have immediately after they are diagnosed with cancer. Patients who have an active role or partake in medical decisions have a sense of power over the situation, which is a huge therapy.

Treatment

Cancer is a complicated disease, and no one doctor is an expert in all aspects of treatment. Developing a treatment plan is a complex task that involves teams of healthcare experts. These experts will give you their advice and recommendations.

In most cases, a combination of treatment options is recommended. This includes surgery, chemotherapy, and radiation therapy. The order of treatment will be determined by the doctor you choose. Depending on your needs during treatment, other professionals might be brought in. For instance, you might require the assistance of a nutritionist for your diet if you are receiving chemotherapy. The assistance of a physical therapist might equally be required, especially if you had surgery.

Social workers and nurse navigators are other professionals whose assistance might equally be needed. The nurse navigator and social worker listen to the patients and their family and their complaints and direct them to resources, including insurance and pastoral care. These individuals, who are mostly provided by the hospital, might equally be leaders of support and discussion groups as well as providing education if needed. For those who will need assistance at home, the social worker and or the nurse navigator will plan for your discharge, transportation, and equipment to be used at home as needed.

Advanced Directives

The cancer journey is one of those journeys that is unpredictable, especially if your disease is in the advanced stage. Having advance directives in place is important in case you're unable to make objective decisions for yourself for any reason. This is very common when patients are depressed, probably because they believe or think the treatment they are getting is not working or they are seriously in pain or mental instability. In such situations, advanced notarized directives are necessary.

Second Opinion

According to the American Cancer Society, one of the most important decisions a cancer patient will make, which will also affect their future, is the treatment decision. Getting a second opinion, both for diagnosis and treatment, is very important for a patient's peace of mind. How are you not sure that some other patient's results or diagnoses were mistaken for yours? As far as your treatment is concerned, seek a second opinion. I had a patient who told me he was more comfortable with one physician over another because while her chosen doctor requested all the medical records, including images of X-rays, CT scans, MRI, and ultrasound, the disqualified physician only used written medical records.

From experience, some patients may be reluctant to seek a second opinion for fear of hurting the feelings of their current doctor. Remember, it is your body, and it is only you and no one else who is feeling the pain. Cancer is a life-and-death disease, and bear in mind that you are just one patient out of the many your doctor is seeing. Thus, hurting your doctor's feelings for what is best for you is the best decision you will ever make in your treatment journey. Equally, bear in mind that you are not the only one seeking a second opinion, and no competent healthcare provider will object to your seeking a second point of view.

Changing Physicians

Changing your doctor for another one is neither uncommon nor unusual. Sometimes, a patient might not be moving along with their physician. Your doctor must give you the maximum attention. Your doctor might be uncaring, passive, or fail to convince you of their competence. If you start having doubts or if any of the above becomes questionable, don't hesitate to ask your physician for a referral to another provider. As a matter of fact, the internet and the American Cancer Society are at your disposal for some of this information. Request all your medical records and also make sure all the records, which include partial treatment, if any, reach your new doctor. Again, you don't want a doctor who will always tell you what you want to hear or a promise of the greatest cure.

Rehabilitation and Recovery

Undergoing cancer treatment is part of the process of the cancer journey. Recovery from the illness and the many side effects from the various forms of treatment is another process that requires a new, expanded team of healthcare professionals. This expanded team might include some of the existing caregivers and more additions, which include specialists in emotional distress, sex therapists, physical therapists for muscular functions, pastoral or chaplain, and coping with life in general after treatment. Most of these other healthcare professionals are still in the hospital setting, which will, therefore, require that the patient still be making hospital visits. On the other hand, some patients will have the luxury of having some of these specialists pay visits to their homes or residences. With the advent of telemedicine, it is easier for physicians to consult their patients while at their homes by video or online.

For those patients who are not sure what to do after treatment, most healthcare providers will recommend outside social workers, psychologists, psychiatrists, and psychosocial and psychiatric nurses who will provide useful information or advice to individual patients or groups. Groups and organizations of cancer survivors, including social workers who are mostly affiliated with hospitals or voluntary organizations, provide useful information as well on how to get some of those resources around your location or community, especially as they have done this repeatedly. Some of this assistance includes helping in placing recovery patients in centers that might meet their needs. Alternative medical practices may be an important resource for those who wish to supplement their care (Living Beyond Breast Cancer; Weiss, M.C. & Weiss, E., 1998).

CHAPTER 10
Metastasis and Recovery

The goal of treatment for any patient is to achieve a cure, but with cancer, that outcome is sometimes difficult—or even impossible—to reach. The initial course of treatment is only successful for a little more than half the population fighting the disease, which implies that these individuals will not have to fight cancer again all their lives. For those patients who are not fortunate to have their cancer diagnosed at an earlier stage when the disease is still localized, it has already spread to other parts of the body or metastasized. The third group is that group of patients who have had their cancer treated, and after a while, it recurs. The duration of recurrence ranges from a couple of months to many years.

Metastasis and recurrence mean that cancer cells have escaped to another part of the body. This might be as close as one breast to another or from the pelvis to the lung or brain, known as distant metastasis. No matter what it is, it does not mean that it is uncontrollable. Again, the conventional modes of treatment, of chemotherapy, radiation therapy, and surgery, will still be used for your treatment. Though the return of cancer may be traumatizing to a patient, effective coping strategies might be very consoling.

Questions for your Doctor

- Is metastatic cancer curable?

- Is there a way to prevent cancer from metastasizing?

- Is metastatic cancer treated like other forms of cancer?

- Does the fact that I have metastatic cancer mean that my children will have it as well?

- What might be my life expectancy?

How Cancer Spreads

Malignant tumors, or cancer cells, spread at different rates and ways, but the progressive steps at which they spread are somehow predictable. Usually, cancer cells spread to other parts of the body either by way of the lymph system or the bloodstream. But no matter how it is transferred to other parts of the body, it is named after its primary. For instance, if your primary was breast cancer, your cancer will be named breast metastasis even if it is now discovered in the brain.

Usually, your oncologist will be able to make an educated guess regarding the likelihood that your cancer will spread or recur based on the knowledge about the type of cancer, the stage at which it was diagnosed, and specific characteristics of the cells identified by the pathologist during diagnosis. While some cancers take a short time to metastasize, others take longer to do so. For instance, breast cancers at the time of diagnosis might already have involved the lymph nodes. On the other hand, patients with prostate cancer might die from something else before their cancer spreads to other parts of the body.

As a tumor grows, a blood supply equally develops to nourish the growing mass. Researchers are currently investigating various ways of assessing a tumor's blood supply. That is why the creation of new blood vessels as a measure of a tumor's potential to metastasize is equally evaluated. They are also trying to determine whether angiogenesis can be used as a guide to predict outcomes and be able to develop new treatment methods (ACS, 2019).

Sometimes, cancer cells spread to areas of the body beyond the original tumors in two ways. The most common is a situation where single cells break away from the initial tumor and enter the surrounding blood vessels. Pieces of cancer cells lodge in capillaries close to the primary site; some cells manage to enter the general circulation, and others enter the nearby lymphatic system as lymph circulates in and out of the bloodstream. These cells that enter the circulatory and lymphatic systems follow the paths of these vessels and often travel to predictable parts of the body. An example is the lungs and liver, the main organs of blood flow, which carry with them cancer cells.

It is also known that cancer spreads to tissues adjacent to the primary site. For instance, a tumor outside the ovary, due to its size, might shed cells that come to rest on the surface of the uterus, which is nearby. Some of these cells will put down roots into the walls of the uterus, and new growth begins.

Secondary Tumors

Secondary tumors or metastases develop immediately when invading cells reach receptive tissues. To ensure the cells' survival, these secondary tumors begin developing a new blood supply in the same sequence the primary tumor took to develop.

Though less than one-tenth of 1 percent of the circulating cancer cells live enough to establish themselves in other parts of the body, about 50 percent of cancers have already spread at the time of diagnosis, depending on the organ the cancer originated from. In some cancers, the involvement of the lymph nodes, metastasis, and secondary tumor are too small to be detected. That is why the removal of the primary tumor during surgery, the oncologist may recommend adjuvant therapy with radiation and chemotherapy, sometimes even when there is no evidence of metastasis. Studies have also shown that chemotherapy and radiation therapy may be much more effective against micrometastases, undetectably small cancers than either treatment is when the secondary tumors are large enough to be detected (Murphy, G.P., Morris, L.B., & Lange, D., 1997).

Bone Metastasis

Bone metastasis is a situation in which cancer spreads to the bone. It is also called metastatic bone disease or secondary bone cancer. Usually, bone metastasis occurs in people who have advanced cancer. This means that cancer has progressed to an advanced stage that might not be curable. Though the progress of bone cancer can be rapid, there are equally slow progressions that can be treated as a chronic condition that needs careful management.

Research shows that nearly any type of cancer spreads to the bone. However, some cancer types are particularly likely to spread to the bone. This includes breast, kidney, lung, lymphoma, thyroid, multiple myeloma, and prostate cancers (Murphy, G.P., Morris, L.B., & Lange, D., 1997). Bone metastasis can occur in any bone, though more commonly in the spine, pelvis, and thigh. Sometimes, bone metastasis may be the first sign that you have cancer, and it can also occur many years after cancer treatment. It is not uncommon for bone metastasis to cause pain and broken bones. In most cases, palliative treatment, which is aimed at reducing pain and symptoms of the disease, is the treatment of choice.

Symptoms of Metastatic Cancer

Usually, metastatic cancer does have rare causes, but when symptoms occur, their nature and frequency depend on the size and location of the metastatic disease. The most common signs include,

1. For bone metastasis, pain and fracture.
2. For brain metastasis, headaches, seizures, and dizziness.

3. For lungs, shortness of breath.
4. For liver metastasis, jaundice, or stomach swelling.

Treatment

Once cancer spreads, it is difficult to control, but the following treatment types are usually recommended depending on the situation. Again, this will be based on your doctor's recommendations.

Medications

Bone-building medications, which are commonly used to treat people with osteoporosis, may also help patients with bone metastatic disease. These medications help to strengthen bones and reduce the pain caused by the disease, thus helping to reduce the need for strong pain medications. These medications might be very helpful in reducing the risk of developing new bone metastasis.

However, based on the prescription or recommendations of your doctor, these medications are administered every few weeks through a vein in your arm or by injection. The oral form of these medications is also available; they are not usually as effective as the IV forms and might cause digestive side effects. The side effects of bone-building medications might be temporary bone pain and kidney problems, and an increased risk of osteonecrosis or the deterioration of the bones (ACS, 2019).

Hormone Therapy

Research shows that for those cancers that are sensitive to hormones in the body, another option is to suppress them with hormones. A good example is prostate and breast cancers that are sensitive to hormone-blocking treatments (Murphy, G.P., Morris, L.B., & Lange, D., 1997).

Hormone therapy involves taking medications to lower natural hormone levels or to block the interaction between hormones and cancer cells. It is not unusual to use surgery to remove hormone-producing organs like ovaries and testes.

Chemotherapy

For patients whose cancer has spread to multiple bones, the physician can recommend chemotherapy. Chemotherapy, which can either be taken as a pill or administered through the vein or both, travels throughout a patient's body to fight cancer cells.

Though hair loss and fatigue are some of the most common side effects of chemotherapy, a patient's side effects will depend, in most cases, on the type of chemotherapy drug administered. For cancers that are sensitive to chemotherapy, chemotherapy may be one of the best ways to alleviate pain from bone metastasis.

Pain Medications

Sometimes, pain medications are used to control cancer that has metastasized to the bones. Some of these medications might be over-the-counter or prescribed by the doctor. These medications are aimed at relieving pain only. The type of medication recommended by a physician will be based on the patient's pain level.

Studies show that it may take time to determine what combination of pain medications might work for a particular patient. It is usually advisable to always inform your doctor about the progress of your pain level. Sometimes, your doctor might recommend a pain specialist to manage your case (ACS, 2019).

Steroids

Steroids are medications that can help to relieve pain associated with bone metastases disease, inflammation, and swelling at the cancer sites. These steroids can work quickly in helping alleviate pain and complications from cancer. Like most other types of steroids, though, these are different from those used by bodybuilders; if used for long periods, complications such as addiction might arise (ACS, 2019).

Targeted Therapy

Targeted therapy is a new class of medications that is now available for some types of cancers. These medications are known to attack specific abnormalities within the cancer cells. Certain cancers, like those of the breast, might respond positively to this treatment. Some researchers explain that HER2-positive can respond to trastuzumab (Herceptin) therapy (Murphy, G.P., Morris, L.B., & Lange, D., 1997).

Radiation Therapy

This is a situation whereby high-energy X-rays are used to kill cancer cells. Radiation therapy is a popular option if a patient's bone metastases are causing uncontrollable pain after using medication. Depending on a patient's situation, radiation therapy nowadays can be administered once or in small doses over a couple of weeks. Again, this is not geared to cure the disease but to help alleviate the pain.

Physical Therapy

Physical therapists work with patients by devising a plan to help them increase their strength and mobility. Usually, physical therapists suggest assistive devices to help patients cope. These devices might include crutches and walkers to take weight off the affected bone while walking, a cane for balance, or a brace to stabilize the spine.

Surgery

Surgical procedures can help stabilize a bone at risk of breaking or that needs repair. For example, if a bone is at risk of breaking due to bone metastasis, orthopedics can use metals, nails, plates, or screws to stabilize the bone. For some bones that are not easily reinforced with metal plates or screws, the doctors inject bone cement into the bone that is damaged or broken by bone metastasis. Sometimes, doctors replace existing bones, an example being the hip bone. Hip replacement is one of the most common types of bone metastasis surgery.

Intravenous Radiation

Some patients have multiple bone metastases. For such patients, a form of radiation called radiopharmaceuticals can be given through a vein. Radiopharmaceuticals use low levels of radioactive materials that have a strong attraction to bones. In this type of radiation, once injected into a patient's body, the particles travel to areas of bone metastasis where the radiation is released. Though this method of treatment can help control pain, some of its side effects include damage to the bone marrow, which can lead to low blood cell counts.

Heating and Freezing Cancer Cells

For patients who have more than one site of bone metastases and who have exhausted every other option, heating and freezing, a procedure that can help kill cancer cells, might be another option.

Usually, during a procedure called radiofrequency ablation, a needle containing an electric probe is inserted into the bone tumor. Electricity passes through the probe and heats the surrounding tissue. The tissue is allowed to cool down, and the process is repeated. Cryoanalgesia, which is a similar procedure, freezes the tumor and then allows it to thaw. Cryoanalgesia is equally repeated over and over again. The side effects of cryoanalgesia include damage to the nearby cells, nerves, and bones, which might lead to bone fractures.

Clinical Trials

Clinical trials are situations whereby medications or treatment methods that are not yet on the market are used. The population has a perception of being used as guinea pigs. Again, these are new treatments that can be used to prevent, detect, treat, or manage bone metastasis.

When Metastatic Cancer is Uncontrollable

The last thing every patient will want to hear is that either their disease is incurable or cannot be controlled. But if you are told your cancer can no longer be controlled, you and your loved ones may want to discuss end-of-life care. Though you might choose to continue receiving treatment, this might only help to shrink the cancer or treat symptoms.

CHAPTER 11

Having Cancer Treatment, The Second Time

Cancer remission may last as long as a decade, but it is not unusual for some recurrences to take a couple of years after the original cancers have been treated. But no matter how long it takes, getting the bad news the second time from your doctor that your cancer is back when you got over with the first treatment is very devastating. Patients are often expected to go through a period of grief, often accompanied by many uncertainties and doubts.

At this moment, many questions are asked. Could it be that your cancer was not well treated the first time, or you did not choose a good doctor for your disease? Most religious patients will go to the extent of asking Why me or saying God hates me. Sometimes, patients of certain backgrounds or cultures attribute it to superstition. Some people express feelings of betrayal by a medical system that, to them, was ineffective because it failed to cure their cancer the first time. Some patients will question themselves if they did something wrong or failed to take proper precautions for the recurrence to occur. It is important as a patient to dispel all these feelings, for you did nothing wrong to be going through this the second time. As most healthcare professionals will tell you, your case is not unusual, and accepting the situation like you did the first time when you were diagnosed with your primary is the way forward.

Additional Care

It is no longer possible at some point to alter the course of a patient's cancer significantly. On the other hand, there should be no point in time that a patient will be told there is nothing we can do about your cancer. Something can always be done to relieve symptoms, ease distress, provide palliative care to ease pain or improve the patient's quality of life. At this point of a patient's journey, the treatment measures initiated are to improve the patient's quality of life. This helps to maintain the best possible levels of emotional, physical, mental, spiritual, and social well-being regardless of how far the disease has progressed.

One of the most important things to be done either by you or those around you is to identify the type of palliative care in collaboration with your physician and to make sure you get it. The patient should make sure they discuss their feelings and needs with their primary caregivers to understand how they want to be taken care of. I had a patient break down into tears because the dose of pain medication prescribed to her was not enough for her level of pain, and nobody was listening to her. She was a drug addict so many years back, she explained, and because she has that in her record, she is not being taken seriously. Normally, your primary care doctor will either refer you to where you will get proper care or will be the provider themselves.

Change in the Course of Treatment

There is no human being who will take it lightly if they must change the course of their treatment from cure to palliative because the curative measures have been exhausted. It is equally difficult for the patient's family and sometimes the doctors or caregivers to come to terms with the fact that all the therapy so far hasn't worked for their patients or loved ones. This conclusion might be based on the following signs, which include the disease not responding to treatment, the side effects from the treatment being debilitating, or the treatment having a detrimental effect on the patient's quality of life.

After concluding that treatment cannot control the advancement of the disease, the next step is to stop the effective treatment and resolve the treatment of symptoms, relieve pain, and manage depression and anxiety. The treatment methods of surgery, chemotherapy, and radiation therapy are usually the treatment of choice, based on what they are trying to achieve, but with the knowledge that it is all palliative treatment and not cure.

A patient may have to make certain decisions regarding this shift from treatment to cure, to focus on palliatives aimed at treating symptoms and pain. Some choices might be difficult to make since they might involve a group of people, such as the primary care physician, oncologist, family, friends, and yourself, due to different points of view. For example, a family member may think that they are giving up the life of a relative to death, while a doctor might want to take an aggressive stand. At the end of the day, a consensus should be reached by all the parties. I had to take a patient's son out for lunch to talk to him about the father's situation, and he was very happy to discontinue the father's treatment. He came back to me two years later to appreciate my input because that was what he needed to make the last decision on his father's case.

Quality of Life

Quality of life has different connotations, and none is universally accepted either by the public or the medical community. But a good quality of life might include things like independence, full functioning of the body and senses, sexual activities, and freedom. On the other hand, quality of life is something personal based on how you want to live your life, depending on your situation. For a patient with advanced cancer, a reasonable quality of life should include relief from pain and other uncomfortable symptoms and the availability of assistance when needed.

An acceptable quality of life might be that which is required for an individual to be treated with respect and consideration that would be expected if an individual were not sick. It may mean maintaining personal integrity and self-worth and a sense of meaning and purpose, such as continued consultation on family and personal issues. In a nutshell, it is having control of a patient's events, or if there is a transfer of authority, at least you have a say.

Care and Communication

Usually, patients who are having palliative care services either have these services provided to them in their homes or hospice. Sometimes, there are intermittent visits to the hospital or specialty units if some specialty treatment is required to reduce pain or treat symptoms. Normally, a patient's primary care physician or community hospital supervises these services. It is also possible that a specialty nurse who is trained in palliative care services will be communicating with the rest of your healthcare team. From studies, patients who have used palliative or hospice services have hope and confidence that they will be looked after without fear of uncontrollable symptoms and pain.

Communication is very important in palliative care. It is easy to talk to providers in your healthcare team about your day-to-day difficulties and needs. Many people with advanced cancer monitor their bodies for signs of anything wrong, in most cases, just because of anxiety and fear. Your caregiver will deal with each worry specially and correctly, keeping you informed of the treatment and other options available to you. Getting a more realistic idea of your future can provide some relief from worries and make a difference in your emotional and physical condition.

It is also not unusual for patients to have a communication problem with their symptoms. This is because it is their first time experiencing such an amount of pain or symptoms. In such circumstances, it is advisable to practice communication, or your caregiver can teach you how to communicate. Sometimes, people learn new ways to communicate. For example, in some families, especially among couples, one person is usually the talker or the communicator. In such situations where the patient is not usually the talker, it may be hard for them to speak for themselves. Specialists suggest that the communicator, if it happens to be the other person, be able to discuss clearly with the person and also be able to discuss with the healthcare team.

Some Common Problems

Until recently, not enough attention was focused on palliative care. But nowadays, palliative specialists are putting a lot of emphasis on what kind of support can best improve the well-being of people with advanced cancers. These concerns include controlling symptoms and maintaining a reasonable quality of life for the patient and their family.

Pain

Pain happens to be one of the biggest worries of people with advanced cancer. This pain could be acute or chronic. But no matter what type of pain it is, it can be controlled. Cancer causes pain if the disease involves the bones, muscles, or blood vessels. Sometimes, this could be a side effect from one or another form of treatment a patient went through while undergoing treatment, like surgery, chemotherapy, or radiation therapy. Pain can steal away your quality of life, leaving you weak, helpless, dependent on others for the simplest needs, uninterested in much of anything, and feeling isolated from friends, places you love, and a lot of other pleasures that might now become rough. No matter the amount of warmth or comfort, you become helpless and dependent.

No matter the level of pain, you don't have to suffer, for your pain can be alleviated. Pain medications have become sophisticated and effective with better delivery systems, new knowledge, and fewer side effects. To alleviate this pain, your doctor can recommend over-the-counter medication or prescription drugs in severe circumstances.

Gastrointestinal Problems
Running stomach and vomiting may be associated with the disease, medication, or treatment a patient is getting to control symptoms. The patient's care team, which at this time is palliative, will evaluate the situation and be able to come up with a form of treatment to address the problem.

Another common effect that is usually associated with pain medication is constipation. A program of treatment to prevent or relieve it should be started alongside the pain medication.

Sometimes, constipation is a common course of distress in patients receiving narcotics for pain, and it should be treated aggressively as the pain itself.

Mucositis

Painful swallowing and a lump in the throat are some common side symptoms of treatment-induced mucositis. This is sometimes characterized by inflamed and ulcerated lining in the mouth, throat, rectum, and vagina. Vaginal mucositis sometimes causes pain, discharge, and or itching. The cause of mucositis can be because of radiation treatment, certain chemotherapy drugs, and yeast infection. Yeast infection is sometimes caused by the suppression of the immune system or by the use of steroids and antibiotics. Common signs of yeast infections are the cheese-like coating of the mouth and vaginal discharge.

Physicians recommend a combination of diet changes and medications as effective ways to relieve mucositis. Diet recommendations include avoidance of spicy, hot, and acidic foods and caffeine, cold milk products, and sometimes sour cream just before meals to coat the passageway to ease discomfort. Avoiding big pills and smashing them before consumption might be helpful. Your doctor can equally recommend non-steroidal inflammatory agents in liquid form to numb the mouth and throat before meals. While oral yeast infection can be treated with anti-yeast medicine, yeast infection of the vagina might respond to vaginal cream or sometimes make a vagina more acidic with vinegar and or warm water douche (Weiss, M.C. & Weiss, E., 1998).

Dry Mouth Pain

Dry mouth is another common effect of medication and radiation therapy. This can be alleviated in a couple of ways. One of the most common ways is cleaning and rinsing your mouth with water every two hours. Other methods include using a room humidifier, sucking on ice cubes, lemon candy, tonic water, pineapple, and chewing sugarless gum (Murphy, G.P., Morris, L.B., & Lange, D., 1997). Most importantly, a patient's mouth should be examined frequently by a nurse or caregiver to avoid infection, which might be caused by a dry mouth.

Respiratory Problems

Sometimes, patients might be coughing and have shortness of breath. When this occurs, the treatment team will evaluate the situation and be able to come up with a form of treatment to treat symptoms. Sometimes, a patient will be given medication to help their cough or medicine to dry up the secretion. It is not equally unusual to put a patient on oxygen. Pain medication like morphine is one of the most prescribed. In hospital situations, a patient is rushed to the emergency room, where they are kept for observation. It is always very important to update your healthcare team on your conditions to enable them to get relief for you.

Loss of Appetite

When patients have advanced cancer, there is a tendency of loss of appetite. Some people develop a dislike for certain foods or reduce their intake of those foods. It is not uncommon for some people to hate meat, fish, chicken, or eggs, and sometimes foods that have even been their favorites. At this point, the nutritionist or the nurse who happens to be part of your palliative care team will be in a better position to give you some guidelines on how to prepare your food or what might help alleviate your appetite. For example, yogurt and cheese can be substituted for meat as a source of protein for those who don't enjoy eating meat anymore. For some people, frequent small-size meals might be more appealing than the big three-course meals. At this point, hot meals are substituted for cold foods. People who don't feel like eating in the morning may be interested in eating in the afternoon. According to studies, poor hygiene is often a big factor in eating problems, which, of course, can be overcome with proper instructions in mouth care. Sometimes, if patients' dentures no longer fit properly, it might impede a patient's ability to eat properly (ACS, 2019).

Constipation

Constipation happens to be a side effect of pain, inactivity, stress, depression, and pain medication. If a patient becomes constipated, there is a high probability that they might develop nausea because the food they eat might have nowhere else to go but retreating up toward the mouth.

Now, as troubling as constipation might be, it is both preventable and treatable. Some of the recommendations to avoid constipation, especially if you are on medications, are to drink lots of liquids, use daily stool softeners, and eat a high roughage diet that includes fresh fruits and vegetables. Once they fill up with water, they help move up the bowels, but if a patient's intake of fluid is limited, they can stay put. If, for one reason or the other, drinking liquids and eating a roughage diet is not helping, some over-the-counter medications like Dulcolax and Milk of Magnesia might be helpful (Murphy, G.P., Morris, L.B., & Lange, D., 1997).

If, at a certain point, the above remedies are not that helpful, then your healthcare giver or physician should perform a rectal exam to make sure the cause of your constipation is not because of impacted stool, which is hard stool, pulling up your rectum. Treatment of unblocking the stool, if the stool is impacted in the rectum, includes softening the stool and taking medications to ease the discomfort. The healthcare provider will, at this point, insert a gloved and lubricated finger into the patient's rectum to break up the hard stool so that it can be passed easily. This procedure is followed by an enema until the patient starts feeling comfortable. Again, work closely with your physician and healthcare professionals, who will give you guardians while watching your blood chemistry, which can be disturbed by excessive bowel stimulants.

Weakness and Fatigue

According to studies, as an illness progresses, a generalized weakness of the patient can make the caregiver and the patient discouraged, believing that nothing is working. Weakness and fatigue can be caused by many factors, which include the progress of the disease, depression, and or certain treatments. Again, understanding the cause of these symptoms is essential in recommending the right or appropriate treatment. Chemotherapy and radiation therapy are some of the treatment types that are most noted to cause a patient's fatigue and weakness. Energy drinks are always helpful. Nausea, pain, and some pain medications are other causes of fatigue and weakness.

Sleeplessness

It is not unusual for patients to have a change in their sleep patterns when they are nearing the end of their lives. The normal sleeping pattern is sleeping at night. However, some patients might sleep during the day when others are around and feel more secure than at night. Once more, it is important to find out the cause of sleeplessness. This can be because of depression, pain, anxiety, or other symptoms. Once the cause is known, appropriate steps can be taken, such as providing pain control, taking sedatives, listening to relaxation music, or keeping night lights, which are some recommendations.

Urinary Retention

This is a condition in which a person's bladder doesn't empty completely, even if it is full, and sometimes the individual wants to urinate. People with this condition are unable to urinate, or they feel frequent urges but only urinate in small amounts. The two types of urinary retention are chronic and acute.

Research has shown that though urinary retention affects both men and women, it is about ten times more common in men than women. It is estimated that the incidence of urinary retention increases with age, especially beginning at age 40 (ACS, 2019). In situations of acute urinary retention, it happens suddenly and can be life-threatening. An individual feels the need to urinate badly, but it is impossible to go. This causes a lot of pain and discomfort in one's lower abdomen. Emergency medical care is the only remedy at this point. Hurry to the nearest emergency room to release the buildup of urine. Again, acute urinary retention is a medical emergency, and to relieve the patient, the doctor will place a catheter into the patient's bladder to let out the urine. This, I think, is the quickest and easiest procedure to solve the problem. If, for some reason, the above method can't be done or doesn't work, a small tunnel can be made in the skin over the patient's bladder and through the bladder wall. A suprapubic catheter, in most cases, can be inserted this way. Emptying the bladder will make the patient feel better right away, and complications will be prevented (Murphy, G.P., Morris, L.B., & Lange, D., 1997).

While acute retention is sudden, chronic urinary retention occurs over a long period. In this situation, an individual can urinate, but the bladder doesn't empty completely. In most cases, people might not even know they have this condition because they have no symptoms at first. It is noted that chronic urinary retention can lead to more complications. That is why it is important to see your physician immediately when you start seeing abnormal symptoms. Some of the symptoms include feeling to urinate immediately after urination, hard to urinate, and frequent urination at night, not because of having drunk a lot of liquids.

Abdominal Pain

The most common type of abdominal pain that cancer patients incur is mostly treatment-related. These are side effects of chemotherapy or radiation therapy. Usually, these types of pain are manifested in the form of constipation, diarrhea, or a complete bowel blockage. Some medications, like antibiotics, can also cause abdominal pain. In such situations, a sample stool is evaluated and might be treated with another type of antibiotic. Physicians will sometimes recommend a low-residue diet. There should be no fruit, vegetables, and limited fiber. Medications like Imodium AD are equally very popular medications recommended by doctors (ACS, 2019).

Other types of abdominal pain include bowel obstruction caused by scar tissue, and sometimes cancer produces crampy stomach pain and bloating, which might be followed by nausea and vomiting. Due to the severity of this situation, immediate evaluation is needed and might end up with a surgeon if the oncologist is unable to manage it. Abdominal pain in the center of the abdomen because of enlarged lymph nodes invading or compressing adjacent organs or nerves is usually common, especially with advanced breast cancer. Liver pain is also a common pain, especially when the liver is distended with cancer. Physicians have used radiation therapy and narcotics to control metastatic disease. Narcotics are either administered by intravenous drip or by subcutaneous pump (Murphy, G.P., Morris, L.B., & Lange, D., 1997).

Forms of Treatment

Treatment of advanced cancer is not out of the same treatment modalities that are used to cure the primary. These include surgery, chemotherapy, and radiation therapy. At this stage of your life, you and your family will have an honest discussion with your doctor, nurse, and other members of your healthcare team on the goals, risks, and benefits of palliative care treatment. In your discussions, the side effects of this form of treatment should be discussed as well. While you may be the central figure in your care, the decision on how to proceed is usually made by the medical team—often with the physician taking the lead due to their greater experience and deeper understanding of the disease. It is important to always ask your doctor about the benefits of your treatment and if there are any risks involved that might make your situation worse.

At-Home Palliative Care

Most people with advanced disease will prefer to be taken care of in their home or that of a family member, especially if there is no likelihood of being cured at a hospital. If offered the opportunity, almost the same number will be interested in any comprehensive program of care at home by all the healthcare professionals they might need. Now, when choosing between being taken care of at home or the hospital, one needs to understand the advantages and the disadvantages of both supportive care programs. This very important decision is left to the patient to make and should take into consideration many factors. What is best for the patient is what we are looking for. There is no right or wrong choice, provided the patient is comfortable with their decision, and it works best for them.

Now, in a hospital setting or freestanding hospice, there is a 24-hour medical service or nurse support. In your own or family home, a patient has a visiting nurse who comes in once or twice a day. In a hospital setting or unit, a patient is separated from their surroundings and family. Usually, in a home setting, the patient is the center of activities. The patient's family is also authorized to carry out some activities for their loved one. No matter what setting you choose, there is a healthcare team responsible for you, headed by a physician.

It is also not unusual for arrangements to be made to take advantage of both the home and the hospital or unit settings. When making this important decision, it is necessary that all the players be consulted. This includes the doctor, nurse, and social worker. Having a good understanding of what each one of these settings entails is very important. Sometimes, families underestimate the challenges involved in care. However, when nurses or social workers are involved, they can provide important information that may impact your care—details your doctor might not be aware of, simply because these professionals often handle such situations more frequently and closely. This might include the availability of some home care facilities, finance, or insurance.

Some Hospice Programs

Caring for the final days of human beings or the sick has become as important as treatment given to them with the hope of a cure. We mostly discuss the quality of life for patients or loved ones, but it is also important to discuss the quality of death and what hospice does. It enhances the quality of dying and provides emotional and physical support in a quality and professional manner, as well as spiritual support. Studies have shown that most workers working as hospice employees have passion for their work to the extent that it has become a calling, not a job. To most of them, it is as if they are taking care of a family member or relative who is in their final days or hours (ACS, 2019).

Professionals and the public alike, according to the American Cancer Society, have come to understand that in the past, people with advanced disease were left to suffer sometimes in isolation when they could have lived well to the end of their lives. It was not unusual for some to express anger and frustration over the belief that pain was inevitable. A variety of special programs have now been developed to take care of terminally ill patients with advanced cancer and their families.

The focus of hospice care is aimed at working with a patient's family to provide medical, psychological, emotional, social, and spiritual needs. Care comes from a continuum of professionals, which includes nurses, social workers, physical therapists, nutritionists, and doctors. If, for some reason, the idea of hospice care does not resonate with a patient, and they still want to receive treatment of chemotherapy and or radiation therapy, it is possible they can stay at their home. This is something like hospice care known as Oncology care, but the level of care will not be as comprehensive as you will get from the hospice.

Some patients will want to stay in their homes till the end of their lives and will not want to go to a hospice, which is for the public. Others who might not be religious will equally resent hospice because since, in most cases, religion is part of the regular hospice, they will prefer their home because they don't want to hear about life after death. Sometimes, some doctors offer end-of-life care services rather than referring their patients to a hospice where they will be able to see their patients regularly, arranging for aide care and hospitalization when the need arises.

Questions for Your Doctor

- Is my insurance going to cover my care either at home or the hospice?

- What is the difference in care between staying in my own home till the end of my life and going to hospice?

- Does your hospital offer end-of-life care?

CHAPTER 12
Hospice Admission

It is always a very difficult moment for the patient, their family, and sometimes even the doctor if every option has been exhausted and the doctor has to announce to the patient that they have about six more months to live. At this point, it appears that illness has taken over, and you have given up medical treatment for supportive care for your comfort only. According to studies, most people are in denial when told they have six or fewer months to live. They always want to try one more therapy, which, in most cases, is never completed before they die. That is one of the main reasons why many people don't seek hospice services. In a nutshell, the numbers are not there. To many people, when the doctor tells them that they have a limited time to live, that might be the very first time they hear about hospice (ACS, 2019).

The admission criteria for hospice may vary, but usually, most hospices accept patients with limited life expectancy, which is six months or less. Home hospice requires that you live within a definite area, have access to a caregiver among your family, friends, relatives, or neighbors, and want to remain at home during the last stage of your illness. This must be a condition if the insurance must cover payment. (ACS, 2019). Hospices, which are reimbursed by Medicare and Medicaid, might have similar admission standards they follow. Starting a hospice requires a doctor's referral, though sometimes one can be referred by a friend, relative, social worker, visiting nurse, or clergyman.

It is very important to have a good discussion with your doctor immediately after they bring it up or when you feel like making up your mind. Usually, doctors and nurses, social workers, and some other healthcare professionals might have an idea of hospices around you that might meet your criteria, including spirituality, if you so desire. Always make sure friends and family members who know you well participate in the discussion. Most importantly, the lead nurse who will be supervising your care has maximum input.

The Hospice Team

A patient's hospice team, in most cases, is an extension of their palliative care team, with probably the addition of clergy and some volunteers. The doctor who refers you to the hospice agrees to oversee the medical decisions presented by the hospice nurse, such as pain medication or intravenous hydration. At this time, the relationship with your doctor changes, and they will still be involved in your care, though from a distance. Most communication with your doctor currently is on the phone. Your visits to the doctor's office or hospital are rare or completely out of the question. Sometimes, the distance between your doctor and the fact that hospitals or doctors' visits are no longer regular might trigger anxiety and depression. It is advisable at this moment to talk to someone who could be your nurse, social worker, or spiritual man. Your doctor could just be a phone call away (ACS, 2019).

At this point, your hospice nurse becomes the primary caregiver who communicates directly with your doctor about your condition and checks your medications. In situations of pain and other concerns, your hospice nurse is the right person to talk to. Another essential part of the hospice is that the facilities always recognize the importance of family, relatives, and friends in the care of their loved ones. Most hospices design patients' rooms to look familiar, like the homes they used to live in.

The Role of Hospice

There is always a misconception that if one goes to hospice, that is the end. Hospice doesn't mean you are sending a patient to die. The hospice recognizes the fact that you are nearing the end of your life, and they make dying as easy and comfortable as possible. Some people feel much better once they join the hospice and start receiving their services. I have heard of situations where patients have been in hospice for more than a year when the prognosis was for six months and went back home.

Normally, hospice workers visit their patients either daily or two times weekly based on need. With the advent of technology, patients' movements have been limited. A patient's nurse is in constant communication with the doctor informing the physician on the status of the patient and medications. Hospice and healthcare workers have the skills to adjust a patient's pain medications to suit their needs in the form of pills, patches, injections, subcutaneous pumps, liquids, or epidural catheters. These workers equally coordinate care with frequent evaluation, treatment of symptoms including pain, and providing comfort to the dying patient, especially if they are on their last days.

At this time of the patient's life, they undergo a lot of anguish, and the hospice workers understand that too. That is why they are trained, in addition to the physical care they give, to provide emotional comfort or support. The role of the family alongside the hospice workers is very important. The patient's children and other relatives will be trained on how and when to give medications, including other practical things like combing or brushing their hair, massaging some body parts like the neck, and telling stories, some of which may distract the patient or make them laugh.

It is not unusual for home health aides to step in for patients who don't have family members or if a patient can't take care of themselves while at home. In situations where a patient is being cared for by the family and, for some reason, the patient needs some professional or additional care, the social worker or lead nurse will be in a good position to give them some information about additional community or county help. The hospice team meets regularly to evaluate each patient's situation and family needs and determines if a patient might need some additional assistance like outings or services.

The Body, Mind, and Spirit of the Patient

Studies and experiences have shown that patients with advanced illness undergo a psychological crisis, leading to a lot of distress that is not easily eliminated. On the other hand, a patient can be relieved of loneliness, feelings of vulnerability, some practical worries, and spiritual and other concerns. In most cases, while people with advanced disease depend on their doctors for cure or palliative care, it is not unusual for them to seek help from other sources, which might help to console or eliminate fear and understanding of certain situations. Sometimes, it helps just to have a familiar face around who makes a patient comfortable and creates a supportive, satisfying environment. Though the team of social workers, nurses, chaplains, etc. might be available at the patient's service, it is also helpful to bring in another face this time, which might not be emotionally entangled to the patient.

At this stage of a patient's life, they need to talk. The hospice team can give the patient the opportunity to openly discuss their feelings, especially those feelings they may not want to discuss with family members for fear of increasing their burden. The team can help to understand and deal with the patient's relatives' discomfort in engaging in sensitive conversations. Respecting the patient's family members who need to talk can be good for them as well because this may prevent later feelings of guilt or unfinished business and start the necessary process of grieving. I remember the last discussion I had with my father two months before he died and how helpful it was for me in grieving and carrying out his wishes.

The Patient and the Family

It is extremely difficult and painful for loved ones who are in an anticipatory grieving situation, but studies have shown that it is a healthy response to advanced illness. Studies also show that unexpressed or unresolved grief can be a source of psychological trouble for family members. Hospice experts have specific criteria which help them detect between normal and dysfunctional grief.

Sometimes, under the stress of grief, strains among family members appear, or old strains may reappear, which might deprive relatives of mutual support, which is most needed at this time, thus causing further pain for everyone. It is not unusual for most conflicts to be alleviated by talking openly about practical matters like property management, settling financial affairs, and how the last medical bills will be settled. It is at this point that most patients who are at the end of their lives will be discussing their funerals, the prayers to be said at their grave, where to be buried, or where they want their ashes to be scattered or kept. In most cases, the hospice team will help facilitate this type of discussion.

Family members may occasionally exhibit unhealthy coping patterns or emotions such as anxiety, denials, abnormal or excessive grieving, or signs of poor adjustment. Professional help provided by the hospice is available to help those in such situations to cope. It might be more difficult for the family of those who are at home for their care. Sometimes, they may think they can't bear the situation or are frightened. However, the supportive or palliative care team is available to give the patient's family all the necessary information or help they might need, including an emotional safety net to listen to their frustrations and concerns.

It is normally very hard for family members to take care of their loved ones who are nearing their end. But from experiences and studies, at the end of the day, those family members are very happy with themselves and the fact that they were there for their loved ones, giving them their best comfort and allowing them to die with dignity. Sometimes, it may be very challenging for family members, especially if they have jobs, small children, and other obligations to take care of.

The most difficult aspect for patients with advanced cancer with young children is how to reveal to the children what is going on with their illness. Counselors, social workers, and the rest of the palliative care team are trained to handle such situations, too. The patient and family members will be guided on how it will be revealed to the children based on age specifics. It is not unusual to involve the school counselors.

Some Life Prolonging Measures

With the advent of technology, patients with advanced diseases can today make choices that were not possible in the past. They can prolong their lives if they desire by making extraordinary decisions. Some of the difficult measures to prolong life include cardiac resuscitation and mechanical breathing assistance in the final days of their lives.

Normally, certain routine measures are known to be carried out in the hospitals during an eventuality. These include the administration of cardiopulmonary resuscitation (CPR) in the event of cardiac arrest unless the patient or surrogates' direction of the Do Not Resuscitate (DNR) order has been issued. To make sure their decisions are carried out in times when they can no longer make decisions, they write advanced directives, which include a living will, healthcare proxy, medical power of attorney, or a document that includes all their wishes.

A living will, which is advisable for everyone to have, specifies what type of treatment an individual does or does not want in situations of terminal illness, like coma, or when you might not be able to state your wishes. A living will is not legally binding, but it communicates your healthcare wishes to your providers and to the person you've designated, such as a proxy or surrogate with medical power of attorney, so they can make decisions that align with your preferences. A healthcare proxy or surrogate, on the other hand, is a legally binding document that indicates who should carry out advanced directives when the patient is unable to do so. It is also known as a medical power of attorney.

Sometimes, these directives are general, but it is advisable to be specific in your wishes. Some hospitals have guidelines and are even required by law to inform patients that they are entitled to advanced directives. It is also very unfortunate that it is difficult to make decisions because of limited information on what might happen if a certain treatment or procedure is stopped. Though there is no confusion about what might happen when certain procedures are stopped, the patient has the right to refuse them. Relatives have the right to refuse certain procedures for their loved ones as well as agreed by medical, legal, and religious groups to whom they have empowered to speak.

Going Home

One would think that with the advancement in palliative and other supportive care services like hospice, people would prefer to end their lives in modern facilities. However studies are showing that the preferred option is to have their last days in their home (ACS, 2019).

Most people will prefer their home because it is comfortable, has familiar surroundings, and, best of all, they are taken care of by family, relatives, and friends. Staying home equally gives one the opportunity to carry on some of the small activities you used to do if they are physically fit to do them. Patients have the luxury of having control of their activities, such as eating when they are hungry, sleeping when one is tired, and not when the hospital or hospice wants them to. While at home, patients avoid some invasive procedures, which are unavoidable when they are confined in a facility. Though the above listed can go a long way to providing emotional well-being to the patient, it is not unusual for so many people to prefer the hospital stay to their home because of the many activities in the hospital.

A patient's homestay may not be as wonderful as it sounds. For one, family and relatives might not always be available when they are needed. Secondly, the resources of the family might not be enough to handle the demands or needs of the ill. Sometimes, it is very stressful, both emotionally and physically, to take care of the sick, which might be very disturbing for family and relatives, especially for those patients whose families had looked up to them for support all their lives. Knowing that there is a doctor around, even if that is not your familiar physician, is very comforting with the notion that if some medical emergency comes up, they will be taken care of. Some home patients might feel frightened because they will not have a doctor at home, especially at crucial moments.

The option of hospice care at home is a good choice to eliminate or reduce some of the disadvantages of home care. It is also important for families to have a care plan in place, including whom to call in an emergency and outline a specific schedule of medication and other professional assistance. This plan should either be a hospital or doctors recommended.

Comfortability

From studies and experiences, advanced cancer is emotionally painful to everyone involved because it entails a lot of work that is not geared toward cure. However, it has been noted that simple remedies, common sense, good nursing care, carefully selected pain relief, and any other thing designed to provide comfort can be relieving to the patient, family members and the healthcare team. Let it be known that palliative care specialists cannot make everything perfect but have a lot of alternatives at their disposal that allow them to make things better for the patient. They will do their best to make sure you are comfortable as you are nearing the end of your life.

CHAPTER 13
Your Job and Health Insurance

In some parts of the world, especially where there is universal healthcare coverage, the issue of health insurance does not come up. If you are sick, you get up, go to the hospital, and you will be taken care of. In a nutshell, in a perfect world, the issue of finance is not a crucial concern on the part of the patient regarding healthcare. Expenses have become a factor in healthcare coverage because of shrinking insurance health plans and sometimes life circumstances that might catch up with those with no life insurance. I have had a patient whose cancer had advanced from stage 1 to stage 3 because they could not afford the cost of treatment when she had her initial diagnosis. Also, some insurance companies don't cover certain modes of treatment. For example, I have had patients come to my department for proton therapy but ended up with regular Intensity Modulated Radiation Therapy (IMRT) external beam treatment because their insurance does not cover the proton therapy that they have desired. The fact that they had a different type of radiation therapy from what they had anticipated does not mean that they were not properly treated. But sometimes the physiology involved may play an emotional role in a patient, a situation you don't want any patient to be in at this time of their life. Cancer treatment can be financially draining both to the patient and their family. That is why information about treatment costs, insurance coverage, and how the family will handle the cost not covered by the insurance needs to be discussed.

You and Your Job

It is rather unfortunate that ill health does not mean that you stop working. One of the main reasons is that your insurance coverage is financed by your employer. Some bosses might be sympathetic and understanding and are able to give their employees flexibility on their schedule and even time off until they get better. Your workplace can be a source of comfort and support, especially if your co-workers are friendly. A colleague of mine was diagnosed with breast cancer, and within three days of her diagnosis, she informed every staff member in the department of her situation. She set up an email group for updates, and every time she had her chemotherapy sessions, which happened to be on another floor in the same hospital, at least three co-workers showed up. Not every person is that lucky. I have had a patient who told me she was fired from work because she could not keep up with work due to her treatment schedule.

The last thing someone should be thinking of at this time is work-related issues. Some of the common concerns facing most patients are whether they will be fired, demoted, or lose their insurance coverage if they can no longer work full-time or have other career opportunities. Some of the above-mentioned concerns, which might be crucial to a patient, can affect their quality of life and some aspects of their existence and lifestyle. A cancer patient who is already traumatized from the disease should not be stressed at this point by job and insurance-related issues.

It is not unusual for patients to have a difficult time at their jobs, both from their employers and other employees. Some employers might have the impression that cancer is an incurable disease and that you will eventually die from the disease. For that reason, they might be reluctant to invest in you either for further training or promotion. They may also have the impression that the patient might constantly be taking time off from work to take care of themselves and be costing the company more, especially if they must be hiring temporary labor. Sometimes, some co-workers are not always helpful. Some co-workers may be resentful because they will have to stretch by picking up the slack or the responsibilities of their sick colleague, which might include longer hours.

Job Application

According to the Americans with Disabilities Act (ADA), employers are required by law to treat all their employees equally and fairly. They should not single out any employee who is either disabled or perceived to be disabled. Normally, during job interviews and on job-related applications, employers are only required to ask job-related questions and not medical history. It is recommended that you don't provide any medical-related history except that related to the type of job you are applying for. Some states may equally extend federal laws to further protect against disability-based employment discrimination (ACS, 2019).

It is possible that when filling out a job application, you might be asked if you have had cancer. This question is illegal; thus, you could skip it. But if questioned why, tell the interviewer that your current health situation qualifies you for the job in question and that your past medical history has nothing to do with the current position. You could go further by saying that you had cancer, but at this point, you are cured of the disease. Some jobs might require medical references, and if that is the case, you provide your doctor's name and contact information. Do not give out any health-related information which is not related to this position. It is advisable not to lie on your job application about your health. This is because there are pools of information about your health all over the place and your employer might discover that you lied on your application about your health, and if this happens, you might be terminated. Being terminated by your employer might be devastating because you may lose your insurance coverage, especially if you have your insurance through your job. For those who depend on their jobs for health insurance coverage, the National Coalition for Cancer Survivors recommends looking for a job with an employer or company that has a large pool of employees where care costs can be reasonable and could cover pre-existing conditions.

Who to Inform About Your Condition

No one will be excited when they get the bad news of having been diagnosed with cancer. At this point, though you have been happily employed, suddenly, you become stressed and start wondering about what to do or where to start. Normally, you are not obligated to tell anyone about your diagnosis either at work or with family except it might interfere with some of your duties like work, which you might need some assistance or flexibility. Now that a patient might not have time at their disposal to waste, it is necessary to inform your boss or employer about your diagnosis. This will enable them to work with you on your schedule or for you to leave. My colleague who had cancer informed everybody in the department immediately after she was diagnosed, and within a week, she already had a game plan. With the input from other colleagues and physicians in my department, it was easy for her to select a doctor who would oversee her treatment process.

Different companies might have various categories of sick leave in their benefit package. Contact your administrator or human resources immediately after you are diagnosed. Probably based on the number of years and your work week, you may qualify for some leave time with pay. If that is not enough, it is possible to work out additional time with some of your colleagues who might be willing to donate some of their leave to help your situation. At this point, honesty and not talking back to your boss is very important. Avoid confrontation with your employer or superiors. Remember, though you may be in a difficult situation, your bosses are equally taking into consideration what will happen in your absence. In some cases, it may be helpful for your doctor to speak with your employer to establish a realistic timeframe for how long you may be away from work.

On the other hand, not all bosses and colleagues might be willing to collaborate with you on your situation. If, for some reason, you and your boss or colleagues are not on good working terms, don't mention to them what you are going through. Some bosses may take advantage of such a situation to make things more difficult for you. After coming up with a treatment plan and time frame with your doctor, you could request your leave to match the plan. You can later ask for extended leave, if need be, for medical reasons, which at this point might be difficult for your boss to turn down. I have had a patient who regretted informing her boss about her diagnosis because she was fired. She realized later she could have worked out a treatment plan that could fit her work schedule without anyone knowing what she was going through. It is also very important to keep records or documentation with dates of any communication on work-related issues you are having with either your superior or your employer. Though you might not anticipate future problems, difficulties may arise for one reason or another, which might require those footnotes.

Health Insurance

Normally, when you are in good health, you might not know what your health insurance covers and what it doesn't. Some insurance providers will not cover out-of-group services. It is rather unfortunate that unless you have a pre-existing condition or an existing hereditary condition in the family, it is difficult to foresee what type of future disease or condition you might find yourself in to be covered for. Most of our insurance coverage is either through our jobs or that of our spouse. When in a situation where your insurance policy does not cover your condition fully, find out if that of your spouse could cover partial bills.

Now, whether you have health insurance or not, if you have been diagnosed with cancer and you are not sure what to do, call the American Cancer Society. The American Cancer Society will be able to give you helpful information based on your situation. Also, there is Catholic Charity, which has recently been very helpful, especially to those who don't have health insurance coverage. Medicare and Medicaid information centers should not be underestimated. You could also talk to your doctor to see if they can give you information on clinical trials. However, the population might have a bad impression of clinical trials or medications that have not yet been approved by the FDA, thus not in the market, but are scientifically proven to be safe for human consumption (ACS, 2019).

No Insurance Coverage

According to statistics, almost a third of Americans do not have health insurance and have difficulty with healthcare costs whenever needed (ACS, 2019). A form of healthcare coverage is important for everybody, though the younger population always thinks they don't need it. Normally, most people get healthcare insurance coverage either through their jobs or that of their spouse. But if you don't have any of the above, explore the chances of having one or what to do with your health when a situation arises. There are government-assisted programs, or you should explore private insurance. Social workers and hospitals are always helpful in assisting patients with no insurance coverage. Sometimes, hospitals have some funds to cover those who can't afford payments for their services.

In desperate situations, you can present your financial condition to your doctor. Some doctors might be able to write off some portions of the bill or come up with a payment plan. The National Cancer Institute might be helpful through its treatment study program. Other helpful sources of funding include the American College of Radiology, and even state representatives can be of great assistance. Be creative and make sure you have exhausted all available resources at your disposal.

Insurance and Divorce

Divorce brings many complications in people's lives, and your health insurance coverage is not immune, especially if your health coverage is under your spouse's insurance. In a situation where your coverage is under your spouse, and you are divorcing, you must do some careful planning. It is not unusual for one spouse to still have health coverage on the other's insurance after divorcing. However, the divorce lawyer should pay extra attention to this clause in the divorce papers.

Relying solely on your former spouse's health insurance can also have its downsides. For instance, if you or your former spouse changes jobs, you might not be covered by their current insurance, especially if they are having their coverage through their new job. Also, co-pays and deductibles might change and are sometimes higher too, to the detriment of the former spouse. Though it might sound good, divorce benefits to the benefiting spouse could become a bad idea at some point.

Life Insurance Coverage

It might be more complicated to buy life insurance if you have a pre-existing condition. The definition of pre-existing conditions may have different connotations for different insurance companies. Some companies may look at someone who has had cancer as a pre-existing condition, though that individual might have been cured of the disease. On the other hand, another company may look at pre-existing conditions as a situation where an individual is currently on treatment for a disease. Whatever insurance company you might be able to get coverage from, bear in mind that the coverage will be expensive. It could be from one and a half to twice the price.

It is important to note that whatever coverage you are looking for, work with an agent who will be willing to listen to you and reason with your situation. Note that you are now a high-risk client, and some brokers may take advantage of your situation for their benefit. It will be helpful if your doctor paints a positive picture of your situation, though most insurance companies already have a negative picture of pre-existing conditions. Be advised that you must speak out for yourself and sound very positive with any broker or agent you are talking to. Do not portray any signs of desperation, and always provide accurate information with persistence.

As earlier mentioned, having life insurance with a pre-existing condition might be difficult, thus, make sure you don't blow your chances. Always make sure you pay your bills on time and encourage your children, who might be younger and healthy, to acquire health and disability insurance at an earlier age. This will reduce their premium with a lot of options.

CHAPTER 14
Living Wills and Advanced Directives

No one can know exactly when they are going to die. But the one thing that is certain is that every one of us must go someday. What we as humans must think about at this stage is whether we can depart with dignity and how our wishes can be carried out when we are gone. We should consider a situation in which, at some point, you can't make medical decisions that might pertain to your condition. From statistics, most people write their wills when they are in good health but also note that you can write and change your will at any moment you want. No matter when you decide to do it, make sure it is written, signed, and notarized.

Power of Attorney

A healthcare power of attorney is an advanced directive whereby someone names a person who acts on their behalf if, for some reason, they can't make decisions or reasonable decisions in case of illness. It can either be called a durable power of attorney or a proxy. Note that choosing a person to act on your behalf in situations of the unforeseen is very important. You might have all the legal documentation regarding your care, but equally note that not all situations are anticipated, and someone must make a decision or judgment at one point about your wishes.

It is necessary to choose a person of your liking who knows you very well. The person you may name could be a friend, spouse, family member, or community member of your choice. It is also advisable to choose an alternative in case your primary choice is not available or unable to perform the duties entrusted to them.

Living Will

Normally, we want to be able to control our destiny at every level, but in situations of incapacity, especially medical-related, you need a living will. A living will is a written legal document that reflects your wishes on medical treatment you will want or refuse to be used to keep you alive. It spells out your preferences on certain medical decisions if need be, such as pain management. Sometimes a patient's consent might be noted or expressed regarding organ donations. For one to determine their wishes, it is important to consider your values. Reflect on your lifestyle, which has been with a lot of independence, and if, for one reason or the other, you are unable to make independent decisions or if life is not worth living at a certain point. Will you want your life extended even when there are no possibilities of your being cured?

At this point, some end-of-life decisions must be made, which, though they may sound easy, are difficult. To help in your decision-making, your doctor might be willing to answer any questions if you have them. Some of the most popular considerations are no cardiopulmonary resuscitation (CPR), no medical ventilation if it's not for cure purposes, no tube feeding except for short periods with the hope of recovery, and will you want your organs or body parts donated upon your death. I had a patient who told me he wants his body donated to science because he has a rare form of cancer, but with the condition that his children be involved in the research till conclusion. Some physicians advise that though you might already have it in your will, always inform your doctor regarding no resuscitation or intubation any time you check into a hospital.

Advance Directive Footnotes

Though oral directives are acceptable, it is important to put everything on paper nowadays. An advance directive should be a written document. In the United States, each state may have different forms which are required. Depending on where you live, these forms need to be signed by a witness and notarized. No matter what your position on end-of-life issues might be, choose an agent or representative who is strong-minded to resist opposing family members' and doctors' opinions. Make it known within your family and circle of friends what you don't want done on your behalf. I have already made it known in my circle of family and friends that if at one point I am in a vegetative state and will become a burden to my children and family for the rest of my life, I shouldn't be intubated.

It is recommended that you review your advanced directives with your doctor, healthcare team, and attorney to make sure the information you provided is exactly your wishes. Also, talk to your family and friends about your healthcare wishes and advance directives. By having this conversation now, you can ensure that your family members and circle of friends clearly understand your wishes and preferences to help your family avoid conflict and feelings of guilt. Other recommendations include keeping your original documents in a safe location and giving a copy to your doctor, agent, or the alternative while carrying a copy with you, especially if you are traveling.

Adjustments on Advance Directives

It is not unusual for people to change their minds about certain positions they have taken. For instance, a story on the radio made one of my patients change his position on donating his organs to science if it could help save other people's lives. It is, therefore, possible that you could change your directives at any time. When you are making changes, make sure you create new forms, distribute the new copies, and make sure the old document is destroyed at all levels. There might be state requirements to change directives, which may vary from state to state.

Before making changes, you should discuss with your doctor and make sure a new directive replaces an older one in your medical file. At every healthcare facility where you have a chart, such as a hospital or nursing home, make sure new intentions replace the older ones. Again, to avoid conflicts among your agents, friends, and family members, inform them about the changes.

Sometimes, it is necessary to review or create new directives due to changes in situation or length of time. A diagnosis of a disease that is terminal and might significantly alter your life may lead an individual to make a change in their will. It is recommended that this should only be done after discussing with your physician about treatment type and care decisions that may be made during the new disease. In situations of a change of marital status, such as divorce or separation, changes can be made as well. Studies have also shown that over time, people's thoughts about the end of life can change. It is advisable to review your directives from time to time to make sure they reflect your current wishes and or values.

Sharing of Assert and Funeral

Families have been torn apart after the death of a family member because of assert and who is responsible for what. That is why everybody needs a will with clearly defined wishes when you are gone. It might be easier for some nucleated families because, in the absence of one parent, the remaining parent takes over the responsibilities of the dead parent, or an older child becomes the head of the family. But with complicated family structures that are coming up recently, and taking into consideration that every state does things differently, and especially if children who might not be biologically related are involved, a will is necessary.

At your death, remember you will not be available to make decisions that will affect your funeral. How will you want to be buried? Do you wish to be cremated, the depositions of your remains, or do you wish to be buried in a cemetery, and to whom do you want to designate certain responsibilities or friends to speak at your funeral service? All of these must be included in your will. I remember Senator John McCain asking former president Barack Obama to speak at his funeral even though they were rivals in a presidential election in which President Obama defeated him. In some cultures, especially those of Sub-Saharan Africa, funerals are end-of-life celebrations that entail heavy expenditures. To avoid embarrassment and confusion, it is advisable to designate and make financial provision in your will properly. Are you the type of person who will want people to donate to your funeral for a course such as brain cancer research or children's education?

Estate planning is an integral aspect of a person's will. Where does your pension go at your death? One's pension is your hard-earned money. This is money you have worked for all your life, and where or whoever is claiming the money at your death should be your choice and not the government's. Every state has different requirements or regulations on who can receive what at your death. It is possible that your spouse could benefit more from your pension if you have included them in your plan even a couple of months before your death. As circumstances change in your life, so should you update your will. Your divorced partner may inherit your pension or assert if they have their name on your pension plan or asset, including your paid-off home, which you wished could have gone to your children at your death.

Over the years, people work so hard, and as some people would say, if people knew what was happening to some of their belongings at their death, some people may be crying in their graves. Certain belongings or claims have been passed over to you by a relative and you equally might have wanted to pass it down to your children or their spouse. The predicament you find yourself in might be that either your children are still young to appreciate the value of what you want to hand down, or you were not moving along with your spouse, and you wouldn't want your valuables to end up in the wrong hands. Specify in your will who will inherit your jewelry or the gold and silver coins collection.

Again, writing a will can be emotionally draining but an endeavor worth taking. It is very important that while you are drawing your will, make sure you give responsibilities to people who don't have any personal interest in your assets or belongings. Note that at any one point if there is any discrepancy in your assets or will, it might end up in the courts. That is why it is important to work with a lawyer who is vested in wills to avoid errors and wasting your money either in estate taxes or lawyer fees among your children after you are gone.

CHAPTER 15
The End of Life Is Here

It is not possible to predict exactly how long you will live, though your doctor might give you six months. On the other hand, everybody with advanced cancer should bear in mind that the end is near. Normally, there might be some consoling stories like remission and recovery, but one should be thinking and preparing for death. Thinking about death makes both the patient and family members anxious. But knowing what to expect, being honest about yourself, answering questions honestly, and being treated with respect gives you a sense of comfort and a measure of control.

At this point, especially for patients with children, before you gather your feelings on how to help your children, you should first find support for yourself and assurances that you will not be abandoned both physically and emotionally by your loved ones and doctors. If a patient is left on their own without someone close to them or living in a new or unfamiliar environment with no friends or family, they may feel insecure, lonely, and desperate. Patients are encouraged to seek support from spiritual leaders, neighbors, and community groups.

Usually, some patients at this point have a crowded and overwhelmed mind with things they thought could take years to deal with. But once a patient begins handling some of these issues and recognizes that they are doing their best to tackle some of them, they might be able to achieve some peace of mind, a feeling they might not have expected. Some patients, at this point, will look at their situation in the religious context as a kind of fulfillment of the prophecy of suffering before dying peacefully.

Facing Mortality

It is always very hard for the patient if they are discussing death, especially if there is no hope for cure or remission. This is a point when a patient has exhausted all the options, has come to terms with death, and does not want to ruin their last days with anything, including treatment. Studies have shown that before accepting the fact that the end has come, patients have looked for alternative measures or medicine and even clinical trials before giving up.

The fact that there is no designated approach to death and how patients face their mortality is sometimes influenced by personality, life experiences, and, in some cases, culture. What might be shocking to some cultures, especially if a prognosis of six months has been given to a patient, is that some cultures look at it gentler and kinder with no denials. Previously, doctors and family never discussed death with their patients, even if they were dying. The patient was protected from the truth, and they did everything to maintain the semblance of normalcy and peace. The fact that a patient was blind to what was going on protects them from anguish.

On the other hand, it deprives the patient and their loved ones of the opportunity to find closure and to say goodbye to one another, an opportunity they might never have again. I remember the last conversation I had with my father, who was merely speculating about the fact that I might never see him again before he died. The discussion helped me to plan for his funeral and carry on some of his wishes. One of his wishes was to take care of his childhood friends who were still alive. Eighteen years after my father's death, I am still carrying on his wishes, and every moment I spend with those friends of my dad is as if it is Christmas to me.

Sometimes, patients deny the seriousness of their illness, and they are convinced that it might be an episode that will either take care of itself or there will be a cure for the disease. I had a patient who was in denial and kept on telling me he was convinced a "White boy" would discover a cure for his disease. These people can deal with death initially, but denial, on the other hand, might be a way of coping and the only way they can handle the situation. Denial, though impenetrable, doesn't protect your family in any way. If you are sick, your family knows, and they want to be able to talk to you about real issues and wishes. Sometimes, they may find themselves in anguish, frustration, anger, and helplessness.

It is not unusual for a patient's family to not want to discuss the gravity of their loved one's situation with the patient. At this point, most doctors will listen to the patient carefully while looking for signs, which will make them know what the patient knows and wants to hear while giving them honest answers.

Dealing with Fear

Many people have never had to deal with death directly or witnessed someone who is dying. The fact that there is a lot of unknown in death makes it very frightening. But the more you know what to expect, the more prepared you are, and the less frightened you will be. In most cases, people always hope for the best, and because of that, they refuse to die, which will happen anyway. Rather than denying dying, it will be advisable to face it, which will help you set priorities in life. Some writers will advise that you convert your anxiety to fear and general fear to specific fear and structure those fears into a series of problems that you can focus on and do something about. It is important always to remind ourselves that we have important things to do that make our life rich and meaningful and to live a full life to the end. Studies have shown that sensitive physicians can be of great help by gathering you and your family together so that you all can talk honestly, and this will help each other to ask questions and come up with solutions before it is too late (ACS, 2019).

Death is known to come in many steps, which include sudden death, a situation whereby at one moment you are fine and the next moment you are gone. Studies have shown that there is no right way to talk about dying, except that any discussion must respect the patient's way of doing things, decisions, and quality of death like the quality of their lives had been. It is always necessary for the patient and the family to develop a sense of understanding at every step of the way. As you are nearing death, bear in mind that no doctor will give you a definite answer on when you will die. Definite answers are believed to be non-therapeutic (ACS, 2019),

It is advisable to know that not all doctors will be there for you when you might need them. This might be because of a couple of reasons. Some physicians may feel they have failed because they couldn't cure you. Others might be too busy with other cases or because of distance. On the other hand, other healthcare professionals who you and your family can talk to, like the social worker, might be very helpful. The involvement of social and support groups should not be underestimated.

What Matters the Most at This Point

People have different things that matter most to them, and at this point in your life, you start getting worried about them if you are not there. For those who have pets like a dog or cat, it is not unusual to hand over their pet to a friend or relative whom they believe can take good care of their pet in their absence. For those who have kids, especially divorcing women, it might be more difficult because they might feel their ex-husbands will now take custody of their kids but might not even have the skills to raise children. They may also have the feeling that their former husbands have remarried with the impression that their ex's present spouse will not be able to take care of her children, or they might not even get along. At this time, former spouses might start talking to each other to discuss their children and get some comfort in that. On the other hand, it is important to put your legal papers together.

Sometimes, a patient might have all types of ideas for preserving things for their children, but it is difficult to go around it at this moment. It might be a good idea for people in good health to think about what they wish to preserve for their children or the future generation and start doing it right now. At this point in your life, try to reach out to people whom you think you could reconcile with before the end, especially parents or children. Some of your kids might never forgive you because you did not give them a chance to participate in the final days of your life. A friend of mine died five days ago, as I am writing, and I'm not sure how I would have felt if I had not spoken to him a week before his sudden death.

Focusing on Comfort and Support

The feeling of being loved by family and friends to a patient who is nearing the end of life is very essential in maintaining their spirit. This can be manifested by holding their hands and talking to them, being available, listening, and sometimes not talking at all has proven to be helpful. On the other hand, some people will want to keep their illness private and wouldn't want to be bothered either by family or friends. That time is precious, and some people will want to preserve their time for the people they love most, especially those worth the emotional energy for sharing and seeking comfort.

Religion or religious counselors, especially people who are religious, are some of the people many patients who are toward the end of their lives will turn to. The church people will make the patient understand that they are blessed and that they may not be able to cure the patient but might be able to heal them spiritually. They give comfort to a patient while bringing to their attention a future that is beyond their lifetime.

It is not unusual for some patients to turn to alternative sources for comfort, such as meditation, philosophical dialogue, and yoga. After a lot of meditation, some people will accept the end of their life because they have reflected on their entire life span and have come to conclude that at the end of the day, they tried and that though they can't still perform some of the activities they could previously do, they can still enjoy their lives.

Sometimes, your family will not talk openly with you, and if this is the case with your situation, especially if it is too hard and the strength and courage are not there to make it work, perhaps it is time to seek a support group. This can be very helpful, especially if you feel well enough to take on something new outside your home. According to studies, people with advanced diseases who are part of a support group are less anxious and depressed and experience less pain. They are generally in better spirits and live longer than people who do not participate in similar groups (ACS, 2019).

It is worth noting that support from other sources, like inspirational books, should not be underestimated. People may find remarkable comfort in books. Joke books shared with a friend or loved ones, especially old jokes, can't be underestimated as well. Humor might be the last thing you think will lighten up a patient's day, but it has proven to be a positive tool for comfort.

Closing in With One Another

As you are nearing the end of your life, the big question now is, how do you manage the passage of each day? Sometimes, you need to connect with those people you care about and be as honest and direct with each other as possible. There might be things you wanted to say but couldn't say earlier in life that had been lingering in your memory. Having conversations or discussions with longtime friends may be assurances that a dying patient's wishes will be taken care of, even after their departure.

Sometimes, it is hard to find the right words. Some people can struggle to say the right thing at the right time, while it might be difficult for some people to say anything at the right time or say things at the wrong time. Rest assured that someone will say something at the wrong time or in the wrong crowd. The wrong remarks can set someone off. A comment like, "You will be alright," might meet a patient in the wrong mood, and this patient might throw it at you. It will be difficult to manage the situation, especially if a patient uses words like, "You don't know how I feel" or "You don't understand what I am going through." Most people are not confronting death, but there is still some value they can share and offer you and your family. The quiet and thoughtful ways that friends and family share and show love with the patient can be beneficial and consoling to the patient's spirit. The last moments with your children should always be well utilized. Tell them how much you love them and that they should think about you though you are no longer with them. Equally, prepare their minds to know that in some situations or circumstances when they think about you, they might be angry, but that as human beings, such feelings will always come up, but that it is ok or normal.

Physician's Assistance

Sometimes, it is difficult for a doctor to inform the patient that the treatment they have been giving them is not working. But even after the patient has decided to stop the treatment, the doctors can continue helping them by always being available, showing care, and being willing to step in and give guidance in making the right decisions. At this point, merely holding hands and listening could be the most effective treatment.

It is important to note that for a patient to get the most help possible from their relationship with their doctor, the two should have a similar approach to care, and the doctor should know how the patient feels about end-of-life issues. Know very well that it doesn't matter if you and your doctor are different in any other way, like sexual orientation. What counts is understanding and mutual respect for each other's humanity.

Preparing Children

Preparing children for what might happen to you may be very challenging. It is easy to handle the younger children because they will always believe you are with the angels or the stars, sometimes looking out for them. On the other hand, older children may want straight answers. Whenever you have an opportunity to talk with your children, make them understand it is one of the stages of life that everybody will follow no matter what. It is possible for children to appreciate what is happening to their parents and can learn some lessons about life.

Children are sometimes more knowledgeable than we think. Parents should not assume that since they don't ask questions, they don't have questions to ask. A couple of things may make them not ask questions. It could be they are afraid, not sure of how to put their thoughts together, or probably feel you don't want to be bothered. Starting a conversation on your situation might open a discussion that you have to conclude by making them understand that your cancer is not their fault and that they are not the cause of your cancer in any way. Allow room for dialogue, and tell your children if they have any questions or concerns about your illness, they shouldn't hesitate to ask you. The younger children may have concerns as to what is going to happen to them when you are with the angels.

It is important to keep talking to your children. It might turn out to be a question-and-answer session. You may be surprised to find that there's little you can say that they haven't already imagined.

Sometimes, children catch conversations, and based on your tone of voice and facial expressions, they might figure out something is wrong, and they may draw extreme conclusions. Though it is important that they know the truth, understand that you do not have to tell them what they don't ask until you become confident that they can handle the situation. The age and maturity of the children should determine the amount of information you reveal to them. It is equally important not to deprive them of hope. Tell them though you might die, there is a possibility that you might get better as well.

It is not unusual for those who love you to be angry that you are dying and someday you are going to leave them. There might be a lot of anger and frustration swirling around the family, which might be directed directly to the dying person as if it is your fault that you are going to die. There might also be guilt from anger, but do everything possible to dispel any lingering guilt. Assure them it is okay to be angry and that it is not their fault you are in the situation you are in right now, and you will never hold them accountable or responsible for anything.

Children's participation after a parent's death is important. They should be part of everything the family does, like mourning and celebrating the life of the departed. Children, as well as adults, need closure. That is why, except in certain circumstances, they should equally be included in the funeral and the grieving process as per the culture or tradition of the family. According to certain cultures, ceremonies are part of the mourning process, and children need all the help they can get for the mourning, too. Whatever the adults are doing should be inclusive to all the family members. It is not unusual for people to feel abandoned after they lose a loved one, and the way adults respond to the loss may help the children to do the same and move on. Note that without help with learning how to grieve, children may carry unresolved issues forward, which might hurt them emotionally in their lives.

Children's inclusion in the ceremony should be an individualistic decision. First, it should be based on the age, understanding, and tolerance level of the child. Going to the cemetery and lowering the casket, even for some adults, is unbearable. If you are not sure a child can handle it, don't take them there, especially the younger children who don't understand what death is, and at this point, they might believe you are doing more harm to their loved ones by cremating, burning or lowering them in the grave. Family traditions for the dead might determine how much children should be included in the process. Cultures that do a lot of singing and spiritual rejoicing might work very well for the children. Gravesite visits, especially in cultures that have memorial days, are advisable to take children to the site on such occasions where they will leave flowers and talk to the departed with sweet words like "We still love you" or "We miss you." Conclusively, who cares for the child after the parent is gone is very important and that is why the substitute should be a caring one.

The Important Issues

At this time, when a dying patient has limited time at their disposal, they may feel compelled to sort through their responsibilities and obligations and set priorities. The patient, at this point, must focus on what is fulfilling, pleasurable and meaningful to them. It might be a tough decision to make on who to see, what to do and what you don't need to spend or waste your limited energy on. It is also necessary to get your affairs in order. This will include re-examining your will and assigning or distributing personal belongings and possessions of value to you.

It is now time to check out pension and life Insurance arrangements for your beneficiaries. For those with young children, it is about time to discuss college plans with them. What is going to happen to the house or property you own when you are gone? Your family and doctor should be aware of your will and advanced directives in situations like coma or cardiac arrest. Sometimes, some responsibilities must be passed on to other family members. This could either be done verbally or written on paper, preferably written on paper, especially if you are not too sure of the individual's full capability. These directives should also include who pays the bills, medical and dental checkups for the children, and other related activities. Managing this significant part of life, even as they hand down activities or responsibilities, might give the patient some measure of satisfaction and even pleasure through this hard time.

Some people find it difficult to accept help from others, and if you are such an individual, you need to calm down or relax your attitude. At this point, you have less energy, so reserve the energy for the most important things and let people help you as much as possible. Know very well that those who love you, like family and friends, are also suffering in their own way and sometimes feeling helpless and unable to make you better. And if some of these members render themselves available for help, take it. Allowing them to come in, in one way or the other, is relieving for them because they believe they are helping your well-being. It is necessary to spend these last days with your immediate family and friends. Talk as much as you can because this might reflect your life, especially to your children, who will live to miss and remember you.

CHAPTER 16
Hope for Cancer Cure

Cancer happens to be one of those devastating diseases that destroys its victims, families, and loved ones. Scientists and doctors are working tirelessly to combat this disease. As a matter of fact, I have heard people compare acquired immunodeficiency syndrome (AIDS) and cancer, and they prefer contracting the former. Their rationale is that AIDS can be controlled through anti-retroviral drugs, while cancer is a lifelong disease that no doctor has been able to contain.

Researchers are conducting studies to discover new forms of treatment to add to traditional surgery, chemotherapy, radiation, and hormonal therapy. Many innovative therapies are beginning to pick up steam to fight cancer and to ideally have fewer side effects than the existing methods. These innovations are aimed at addressing the issues of aggressive treatment, recurrence, and side effects. Some of the below cancer research breakthroughs are giving us hope for better therapies and preventive methods with fewer side effects.

Immunotherapy

Immunotherapy is a class of drugs that harness the body's immune system to attack cancer. It is aimed at reinforcing the existing potential of our immune system. Some experts think that the upgraded or newer immunotherapy drugs may have the potential to fight cancer more effectively and with fewer side effects than other traditional approaches. In a nutshell, through immunotherapy, researchers are exploring new ways to deactivate the protective system of cancer cells.

One such advance is the Chimeric Antigen Receptor (CAR) T-cell therapy. In this type of treatment, immune cells called T cells are removed from a patient's blood, modified in the lab to attack malignant cells, and then returned to the body, where they look for and destroy cancer cells. Though most of these immunotherapy drugs are still in labs and pharmaceutical companies, the future of cancer treatment is bright. On the other hand, certain types of immunotherapy drugs will not work for everybody. This might be because of hereditary genes of the patient or environmental factors. The hope, as some scientists will say, is that some of this new information or findings can lead to new drugs and interventions that can expand the fraction of patients responding to these new immunotherapies (NCI, 2022).

Targeted Therapy

Targeted therapy drugs are known to attack a specific feature or a target in cancer cells while leaving the surrounding healthy cells untouched. Studies show that there are far more known targets than targeted treatments, but pharmaceutical companies and clinical trial centers are coming up like mushrooms with bright ideas.

Combining drugs with different targets will result in the treatment that will finally put a dent in cancer like it is doing in AIDS. Research is showing that combining the increasing number of cancer therapies has so far proven difficult due to the limited number of possible combinations. However, new approaches in the field of systems biology that use computer models to predict therapy effects are promising to cut through the complexity. They will be able to deliver effective combinational therapies in the future. Some papers state that this type of treatment can be loaded to treat invasive carcinomas such as endometrial and breast cancers. This technique is believed to replace chemotherapy in the future. (NCI, 2022).

Starvation of Tumors

A novel approach to destroy cancer is by starving the cancer cells. Studies are ongoing to prove multiple ways of cutting cancer cells' nutritional supplies. Stopping the glutamine supply is noted to be one of the effective ways of using this approach. It will maximize oxidative stress and induce cell death. It is also noted that blocking the supply of vitamin B2 can halt cancer stem cells. This strategy can, therefore, help to avoid the toxic effects of chemotherapeutic agents (NCI, 2022).

Fluid Biopsy

Usually, during cancer treatment, biopsies are needed many times before the end of the treatment. This is a means to sample the changing tumor to come up with a new treatment strategy. This could be a challenge for the patient and the doctor with the current invasive biopsy techniques. Fluid biopsy extracts cancer cells from a simple blood sample. This is predicted to be one of the next big breakthroughs in oncology (NCI, 2022).

According to the National Cancer Institute, it is noted that some major cancer centers are exploring Deoxyribonucleic Acid (DNA)-based liquid biopsies where a patient's blood is analyzed for types of tumor material such as mutated DNA, Ribonucleic Acid (RNA) or proteins. Predictions are that someday people could be diagnosed with cancer earlier than they would be by traditional methods such as imaging tests like the MRI, CT scan, X-ray, etc.

Like most new technology, there are some concerns about using this technology. Liquid biopsies could show false positives. This means that they could indicate a potentially cancerous DNA mutation when none exists. Sometimes, someone may have mutated DNA and never develop cancer. Though still in the developing stage, these types of tests are believed to be the technology of the future for early cancer screening, especially for high-risk people like those who have a history of cancer in their family. It is possible that it could be used as a pre-screening technique to be followed by some other traditional method, like PET or MRI.

On-the-Spot Cancer Diagnoses

Cancer diagnoses must be early and accurate to achieve good results. Many cancer types cannot be detected early enough while others are detected in time but not treated severely. This notion requires great healthcare facilities, new diagnosis techniques, and proactive patients.

According to studies, an intelligent surgical knife (the iKnife) was developed by Zoltan Takats of Imperial College London and works by using an old technology where an electrical current heats tissues to make incisions with minimal blood loss. Using the iKnife, the vaporized smoke is analyzed by a mass spectrometer to detect the chemicals in the biological sample. This will help allow real-time identification of malignant tissues. It is predicted that surgeons will love this knife, which can significantly reduce the length of operations in oncology (Informed Decisions; Murphy, G.P., Morris, L.B., & Lange, D., 1997).

Cytotoxic Therapy

This is a situation whereby tumor cells' modulation changes the cancer cells' biology so that they become weak and die. Cytotoxins are some of the agents used for this approach. One of the best-known cytotoxins in this category is tumor necrosis factor, a toxin secreted by activated macrophages to selectively kill tumor cells, principally by interfering with the blood supply.

According to the National Cancer Institute, certain agents make the antigens on cancer cells more recognizable to antibodies or sometimes make them stickier so that antibodies bind to them more easily. On the other hand, there are situations where other compounds interfere with a cell's ability to metastasize.

Monoclonal Antibodies

Since monoclonal antibodies were developed more than forty years ago, the idea of a magic bullet or a single agent to destroy cancer without harming the surrounding tissues seemed close to reality (ACS, 2019). These laboratory-made antibodies are manufactured or cloned from the same living parent cell and are designed to link up with matching antigens on the surface of particular cancer cells.

These manufactured antibodies can be made to react directly against cancer cells or to carry radioactive molecules or anticancer drugs to them. Pathologies use monoclonal antibodies in the laboratory to test blood and tissue samples experimentally by radiologists to highlight sites of metastasis so they will be noticeable on medical or radiologic images.

Monoclonal antibodies are also noted to play a key role in bone marrow transplantation. An example is a situation whereby cells harvested from donated marrow are mixed with antibodies in the laboratory and prepared to seek and destroy disabled T-lymphocytes that will normally lead to rejection of the marrow. At this juncture, the marrow is now free of the T cells and can be infused into the host. Though experiments are still being conducted, studies show that the greatest potential for monoclonal antibodies is for cancer treatment (NCI, 2022).

Obstacles to Monoclonal Antibodies

According to the National Cancer Institute, studies have shown that success with monoclonal antibodies has been elusive for a couple of reasons. Some cancers may produce cells whose surfaces are studded with more than one type of antigens, an example being small-cell lung cancer. In such cases, the specificity of the antibodies works against the therapeutic process since different monoclonal antibodies will be needed to destroy this type of cancer cell.

Secondly, once monoclonal antibodies bearing anticancer drugs are injected, they must hold their strength long enough to reach their target. It is noted that if released too soon, toxic or radioactive molecules can enter the circulatory system and destroy healthy tissues or cells. Sometimes, on the other hand, the antibodies may successfully bind to the antigen but fail to release its toxic material.

Cancer cells are also noted to defend themselves in various ways against attacks by monoclonal antibodies. They are sometimes noted to shed their antigens, thereby leaving monoclonal antibodies without an invasive site. Cancer cells may sometimes secrete a blocking factor that coats their antigens that disguise their appearance.

Side Effects of Monoclonal Antibodies

Sometimes, there is pain or inflammation at the injection site. It is also noted that many people experience flu-like symptoms like fatigue, fever, chills, headache, nausea, and vomiting. There may be a decrease in blood pressure, weight gain, and swelling due to the accumulation of body fluids that have shifted from other parts of the body. It should be noted that the side effects may depend on the targets of the antibodies. Prime examples of monoclonal antibodies aimed at colon cancer are sometimes known to cause diarrhea, while those used against a blood disorder may cause a decrease in some white blood cells (NCI, 2022).

Some people also experience allergic reactions such as cough, skin rash, and wheezing. In severe cases, potentially fatal allergic reactions known as anaphylaxis produce a drop in blood pressure, difficulty breathing, swelling, and severe rash. Studies have shown that the risk of allergic reactions increases with each injection because the body forms antibodies against the monoclonal antibody itself (NCI, 2022).

According to the National Cancer Institute, it is recommended that those receiving monoclonal treatment be in a facility equipped with resuscitation equipment in case of allergic reactions. Patients must be observed closely for at least an hour after the injection. Heart and lung functions should be checked frequently, including blood tests, scans, and routine response monitoring of the body's response to the treatment.

Side effects and problems associated with this form of treatment are a huge factor in several areas of research. An example is that many monoclonal antibodies used today are produced from mouse cells because monoclonal antibodies from human cells are less reliable as antibody factories, though they have less risk. It is recommended that more effective monoclonal antibodies be developed in the future while also figuring out ways to prevent tumor cells from changing their antigens, which will facilitate the monoclonal antibody's ability to bind to their targets. A combination of monoclonal treatment methods with other agents, such as interferon, will increase the success of the approach. The treatment of cancer in which tumor-specific antigens can be identified, such as certain forms of leukemia and B-cell lymphomas, has the greatest potential (NCI, 2022).

Interleukins

Interleukins are a subset of a larger group of cellular messengers called cytokines, a modulator of cellular behavior. They are one of the producers of lymphocytes, a hormone-like substance that activates several components of the immune system. Individual interleukins are identified by numbers, such as Interleukin IL-2, which can be mass-produced using genetic technology, which is one of the first approved biological treatments for kidney cancer. Studies show that a certain percentage of patients taking this form of treatment have their tumor reduced in size, and there is also an equal chance of the tumor disappearing completely. It is noted that IL-2 has some success in correcting T-lymphocyte abnormalities in patients with AIDS (NCI, 2022).

Interleukins are involved in the regulation of a variety of physiological and pathological conditions, such as normal cell growth, recognition, and elimination of pathogens by immune cells. They are important in stimulating immune responses such as inflammation. Treatment with IL-2 might be complicated, toxic, and expensive. A typical protocol for a disease like renal cancer is given intravenously four times a day for four or five days. A second cycle begins a week later. According to studies, IL-2 can also have some anti-inflammatory effects, which further complicates its characteristics (NCI, 2022).

Combined Therapy Mechanism

A combination of IL-2 with lymphokine-activated killer cells is one of the areas of focus. With one of these procedures, T cells are removed from the blood and grown in the lab along with IL-2. The interleukins stimulate the T cells to release Cytokines such as tumor necrosis factor and gamma-interferon. These stimulated cells, which are known as lymphokine-activated killer (LAK) cells, are reinserted intravenously. As soon as these LAKs are inside the body, they start destroying a wide variety of tumor cells. More often, to enhance the LAK activities, an additional dose of IL-2 is recommended to be given at the same time (NCI, 2022).

According to the National Cancer Institute, administering IL-2 in low doses as quickly as possible and giving it for long periods after the infusion of LAK cells helps reduce the risk of life-threatening toxic reactions. Studies have shown that IL-2 and LAK cells produce, to a lesser extent, some response in 15 to 30 percent of people with renal-cell carcinoma and up to 40 percent in those with melanoma. Treating gliomas with this method has also shown some good responses.

Interleukins are not stored within cells but are instead secreted, often rapidly, in a short space of time, usually in response to a stimulus. Once interleukins are produced, they travel to their target cell and bind to it via a receptor molecule on the cell's surface. These interactions trigger signals with the target cell that end up altering the cell's behavior. The response of a particular cell to these compounds depends on the ligands, specific receptors expressed on the cell surface, and the particular signaling cascades that are activated.

Side Effects

Treatment with IL-2 is noted to carry a considerable risk of serious side effects. This type of treatment is advised to be administered in a hospital with an Intensive Care Unit facility or emergency physicians available. It is advisable that blood pressure, urine output, and the patient's breathing be monitored for a few days after administration.

Potential life-threatening reactions include arrhythmias, angina, myocardial infarction, infections, neurological problems, and gastrointestinal bleeding. Sometimes, people have kidney failure, and when this happens, they require dialysis. It is noted that about 2 to 4 percent of patients who have kidney cancer and are administered this type of therapy die (NCI, 2022). The good thing about interleukins is that most people recover from this form of treatment.

Capillary leak syndrome, a situation whereby fluid escapes from small blood vessels, resulting in swollen tissues, is of great concern. A patient will exhibit symptoms that include rapid weight gain, a drop in blood pressure, and difficulty breathing. If left untreated, the syndrome can cause kidney failure and or respiratory arrest (NCI, 2022).

There are some minor consequences, such as skin rashes and flu-like symptoms of chills, fever, nausea, and vomiting. Malaise and fatigue are also associated with IL-2 therapy and are exhibited by most patients. It is advisable for people who are receiving this therapy to seek counseling and nursing care.

Hormones and Growth Factors

Though growth factors help normal substances to grow, they are also known as colony-stimulating factors or hematopoietic factors. The Food and Drug Administration (FDA) has so far approved two of these factors for cancer treatment. These include those that stimulate the bone marrow to make normal cells and those that act as anti-cancer agents (NCI, 2022). The following are some of them;

Thymic Hormones

The thymus is known to be the master control center of the immune response in many ways. Most researchers believe that supportive treatment using hormones to regulate this gland may be of great value in preventing infections.

The role of two compounds is being explored for clinical trials. One of them is thymosin fraction 5 and thymosin-alpha-1, used in patients of all ages undergoing cancer treatment and in those with HIV infection who don't have full-blown AIDs or other immunocompromised disease (NCI, 2022).

Mild side effects are associated with thymic hormone treatment; there could be inflammation at the injection site. There might be some toxic reactions, but they are very rare. Studies have shown that those taking these hormones have their sense of well-being improved and are able to function in their daily lives. Most patients' infection rate drops, they regain lost weight, and in some people, there is an improvement in chronic conditions such as arthritis (NCI, 2022). Like every other cancer treatment, the patient and or their family is advised to have a discussion with their doctor.

Erythropoietin

Erythropoietin, in its short form EPO, is one of the first growth factors to be synthesized and possibly best known. This hormone, which is partially produced by the kidneys, causes red blood cells to develop and stimulates their release from the bone marrow. It was approved in the late 1980s for use in chronic kidney disease (NCI, 2022).

In most cases, patients with advanced kidney failure who cannot make enough erythropoietin and are on dialysis may require a blood transfusion. The injection of erythropoietin helps maintain a healthy level of red blood cells and can help eliminate the need for transfusion (NCI, 2022).

According to the National Cancer Institute, though this form of treatment does not directly address the cause of kidney failure, it is known to offer valuable support to improve the quality of an individual's life. The replacement of erythropoietin also helps to reverse the anemia that often results from chemotherapy with cisplatin. It is noted that people who are receiving erythropoietin report a sense of well-being and higher energy level, which enables them to live longer.

Vaccines

Vaccines are gaining traction worldwide because they have proven effective in preventing infectious diseases. Cases in point are diseases such as polio, smallpox, and, most recently, COVID-19. For cancer, scientists are struggling to come up with a vaccine designed to immunize patients against their own disease or tumors.

Cancer vaccine development and testing are ongoing worldwide, though with mixed results. Scientists are conducting clinical trials with constant improvement in the outcomes. Melanoma vaccines are noted to be one of the most active areas of involvement (NCI, 2022). Some small studies indicate that some combination treatments employing a vaccine prolong survival time. In some cases, vaccines will be combined with interferon treatment.

Tumor Necrosis Factor (TNF)

TNF is secreted by cells, including macrophages, which kill tumor cells directly. It enhances the effectiveness of some anti-cancer drugs and also boosts interferons and interleukins. Some researchers believe this growth factor shrinks tumors, thus enabling other treatments that activate the immune system to destroy cancer cells more effectively. According to the National Cancer Institute, there is some evidence that injecting tumor necrosis factor directly into Kaposi sarcoma lesions, which are related to AIDs, will provide some benefits.

Usually, the route of administering TNF is determined by the type and severity of the negative or adverse reactions. It is noted that intravenous infusion produces long-lasting and more severe shivering and fever. It is also observed that after injection under the skin, fatigue is more common and severe, and skin rash is more likely (NCI, 2022).

The skin side effects of TNF are sometimes noted to resemble those of other biological treatments, which are flu-like symptoms in nature, such as chills, fever, headache, and inflammation at the injection site. People with abdominal disease may sometimes experience nausea and vomiting. Other common effects of a lesser degree include a change in blood pressure, rapid heartbeat, fatigue, and mild chest discomfort. The good news is that people who receive daily doses of TNF are able to tolerate the side effects well enough (NCI, 2022).

Research is being conducted daily on the functioning of the immune system and cell multiplication and coordination. Researchers are also learning about the relationship between humans, the host, and the disease and how tumor cells and the immune cells interact. Studies show that there are countless opportunities for therapy aimed at improving the body's ability to fight the disease. Based on clinical trials, cells removed from the body can be inserted into genes programmed to produce more TNF and later reinjected into the body. Based on conducted studies, there is no doubt that biological therapy is promising to help solve the cancer problem (ACS, 2019).

CHAPTER 17
Bone Marrow Transplant

The removal of bone marrow from one person and the return of blood-forming cells to the same person or somebody else is what is often referred to as bone marrow transplant (BMT). This procedure is sometimes called peripheral stem cell transplantation. BMT was developed for people whose defective marrow caused conditions such as aplastic anemia, but today, it is being performed mostly for cancer patients (Murphy, G.P., Morris, L.B., & Lange, D., 1997).

Bone marrow is the tissue within the cavities of bones that contains fat and blood-forming tissues. Healthy bone tissues are noted to replenish the blood supply constantly and are essential to our well-being. BMT is not a treatment, but it allows patients with cancer to undergo other aggressive forms of treatment, such as chemotherapy and radiation therapy.

For patients who undergo chemotherapy after a BMT, there are usually two ways to approach this. There is the high-dose chemotherapy approach. With this approach, the protocol mostly starts with initial standard-dose chemotherapy. If the patient responds well, they will now proceed to high doses of chemo either with the same agent or with other drugs. Another less common approach is getting high doses of chemotherapy right away after harvesting the bone marrow. It is not yet very conclusive that BMT is very effective (ACS, 2019). Secondly, BMT can be life-threatening as well. It is necessary to have a full discussion of the side effects of the procedure as well as alternative methods of treatment with your doctor.

Some patients undergo radiation treatment after BMT. This is usually total body radiation. When a patient is undergoing this form of treatment, they are usually hospitalized or inpatients. This is because, first, the patient usually has a weak immune system, so they are trying to minimize infection. Secondly, in case of any complication, it can more easily be corrected in a hospital environment than at home.

Medical Development

Scientists in the 1950s discovered that the red bone marrow drawn from one person could be infused into another person, and the immature cells, also known as stem cells, would shortly begin to produce normal blood cells. By doing this, stem cells in the bone marrow that have been destroyed could be replaced and begin turning out oxygen-bearing red blood cells, infection-fighting white blood cells, and platelets, which assist blood clotting (Murphy, G.P., Morris, L.B., & Lange, D., 1997).

With the development of techniques that allowed precise genetic matching of bone marrow recipients and donors in the 1960s, BMT became a vital tool in the treatment of some blood cancers like leukemia. By the 1980s, BMT had become a viable tool in the treatment of other forms of cancer (Murphy, G.P., Morris, L.B., & Lange, D., 1997). Techniques that enhance the recovery process, such as using new drugs to boost cell production, are making BMT safer and shortening hospital stays. Studies are underway for outpatient care for part of the procedure.

BMT, though promising, requires a tremendous investment of time, energy, and patience. It also demands bravery because of the risks involved, which include rejection, death, and sometimes long-term consequences. The success of BMT is higher in the younger patient age group and if the disease is still in the early stages.

Candidates for Bone Marrow Transplant

Though BMT might be a good method for cancer care, in some cancers, particularly those involving blood cells, a bone marrow transplant is used to attack the malignancy directly. Leukemia, multiple myelomas, myelodysplastic syndromes, non-Hodgkin's lymphoma, and Hodgkin's disease are among the diseases that are suitable for a bone marrow transplant (Wess, M.C. & Weiss, E.,

1998). It is also good to note that some solid tumors, such as cancers of the lung, breast, brain, and testes, may also qualify for bone marrow transplant (Murphy, G.P., Morris, L.B., & Lange, D., 1997).

Bone marrow transplant is, however, noted to be a rescue procedure replacing destroyed bone marrow tissues when extremely high doses of chemotherapy drugs or radiation therapy have been used. Some studies are still in the experimental stages, especially in the treatment of some cancers, such as breast and lymphocytic leukemia (Weiss, M.C. & Weiss, E., 1998).

Note that patients have absolutely no bone marrow for some time during the transplant, and the number of circulating blood cells takes a while to return after the marrow is transplanted. Candidates must be strong enough to withstand a variety of complications that might arise. Candidates should also be able to endure aggressive treatment. That is why physicians and transplant centers properly screen candidates.

Searching for a Donor

Studies have shown that more people are volunteering to become donors of their bone marrow. This is because more people are learning about the success of bone marrow transplants. So many people have registered to become donors from statistics, but the chance of having a match is not that easy. That is why most people will begin with family members, especially siblings, whose bone marrow could be a match. It is usually an expensive venture, even among family members. This is because travel is expensive, especially if relatives are scattered either all over the world or in different parts of the country.

In some situations, a family member whose marrow matches the patient's is not that candidate's favorite in the family, which, of course, can create another obstacle. Though in situations of need, most relatives wouldn't mind, are you comfortable asking for such a favor from someone you haven't spoken to for a long time, due to one reason or another? Sometimes, a relative might refuse to be a donor, which, of course, might create resentment and anger. It becomes even harder to find a donor, especially if a candidate was adopted. Compared to many years back, with computers and large marrow banks such as the National Bone Marrow Donor Program in the United States, it is easier to find donors. Some communities have made it easier by hosting donor parties.

Steps of Bone Marrow Transplant

The steps of bone marrow transplant are almost similar, though they might vary slightly based on the purpose. Standard-dose chemotherapy is one of the steps. The purpose of standard-dose chemotherapy is to eradicate cancer and test the cancer's response to chemotherapy (ACS, 2019). This process, which takes place in specialty conditions, is either done in an outpatient or inpatient facility.

Harvesting bone marrow is aimed at the removal of immature immune cells and mature cells before high doses of chemotherapy damage them. This process usually takes place in the operating room. After the procedure, the patient is taken to the recovery area for observation and later released the same day or the day after. Harvesting peripheral stem cells has the same purpose and process as harvesting bone marrow. While harvesting bone marrow takes place in the operating room, peripheral immature stem cells and mature immune cells are collected by apheresis as an outpatient procedure. Each apheresis takes about two to six hours.

Another crucial step is processing and storing immune cell samples. This process filters the immune cell mix. Cancer cells are purified, and samples are frozen. Liquid nitrogen freezers in hospitals or other appropriate facilities are conducive environments for storage.

Normally, high-dose chemotherapy effectively eradicates cancer cells, which is not possible at lower doses. This process typically occurs in specialized isolation rooms within hospitals, as the patient's critically low blood counts require strict infection control to minimize the risk of illness. Sometimes, a patient might go home with special precautions, but this only takes place when a patient's counts are above the critical level.

The last step is restoring the immune system with reinfusion of the immune cell mix. Because of possible complications, this is mostly done in the hospital, which has enough personnel in case of an emergency.

Testing the Donor

A human leukocyte antigen (HLA) is a technique that has improved matching tissue typing. HLA cells on protein surfaces help cells recognize foreign substances. They play a vital role in the immune response and the acceptance of the transplant. Studies have shown that the better match of the donor and recipient's antigens, the less likely the marrow will be rejected and the fewer complications during the process. Usually, when a match is made, the donor is tested for HIV, hepatitis infections, and other diseases that the transplant might spread.

The donor has an important responsibility. It is always important for the donor to understand fully the scope of the undertaking before agreeing on the procedure. Apart from the fact that there is a lot of pain encountered during the extraction, the donor is usually on call, waiting for the best time their marrow will be removed, which is based on the recipient's blood count and general health.

Experience has shown that donors are happy that they can help, while some worry that their marrow might not be good enough to cure the recipient. Some donors also feel responsible for the success or failure of the treatment, as if they have control over anything. It is also noted that some donors, though hesitant to say it, feel ignored throughout the whole process because all the attention is focused on the recipient (NCI, 2022).

Types of Bone Marrow Transplants

Bone marrow transplants are categorized according to the source of the marrow, which, of course, indicates how close a match they are.

Syngeneic transplants are the most compatible bone marrow transplants. They use the bone marrow of identical twins. There is no risk of rejection in a syngeneic transplant because the twins' human leukocyte antigens (HLA) are a perfect match; therefore, it is perfect (NCI, 2022).

Allogeneic transplant is a type of bone marrow donated by a person chosen through the human leukocyte antigen typing process. The better the match is, the less the risk of rejection will be. Studies show that siblings are always a closer match than parents and are more likely to be compatible than other family members. The best matches, in a nutshell, are those from the same ancestry. Research has shown that it is difficult to find a match for people belonging to minority populations, such as those of Asian and African descent. This is because fewer minority groups are in the pool currently. Efforts are being made to recruit minorities and encourage them to become donors so the shortage or scarcity may be overcome in the future (NCI, 2022).

Autologous transplant is a form of bone marrow transplant, which is the removal of bone marrow from the person with cancer before treatment and its return to this individual after treatment of either high doses of chemotherapy or radiation therapy or a combination of the two. Usually, during the couple of weeks that the therapy is underway, the marrow cells are frozen. There is no risk of rejection because the marrow is the person's own, but there is a chance of reintroducing cancer cells that might remain in the marrow. To minimize this risk, some laboratories treat the marrow either with chemotherapy, special antibodies, or other substances before reinfusing, a process known as purging (NCI, 2022).

According to the National Cancer Institute, autologous transplants are sometimes still considered experimental but are used for forms of solid tumors like breast cancer. Some recent developments include the banking of umbilical cord blood obtained when a baby is born for use later should the child need high doses of either radiation therapy or chemotherapy. This precautionary measure will be most appropriate in a situation where there is a history of cancer in the family. Otherwise, it might be a waste of resources to be preserved for so many years.

A variation of bone marrow transplant, which is the harvesting of blood stem cells, is under study (NCI, 2022). In this situation, immature blood cells are withdrawn from the recipient's blood and later stimulated in the laboratory with natural chemicals called growth factors to produce enough stem cells for transfusion.

Risk Associated with Bone Marrow Transplant

Usually, it takes an average of one month for your transplanted stem cells to start making new cells to reach a critical defense guard. At this point, they are just about able to protect the patient from infection. For some patients, full recovery of the immune system can take many months. Side effects from bone marrow transplant can sometimes be very severe and usually depend on which of the chemotherapy agents and blood products are used. The biggest risk is a severe infection that can result in death.

Studies show that the high risk of life-threatening infection continues if the immune cell count remains below 500. Until the transferred stem cells have recovered to about 1500 or above, the patient's body's defense is still vulnerable (NCI, 2022). Your doctor may prescribe special growth factors to stimulate faster recovery and proliferation of the stem cells. Transfusion of someone else's immune cells may be necessary. Antibiotics are commonly used at the slightest notice of infection, and isolation from sources of infection is usually the standard policy (NCI, 2022).

Infection

Since the bone marrow is part of the patient's body's infection-fighting system or immune system, if it is taken, the system is weakened. When an individual's system is weakened, the body cannot protect itself as well against germs. Most of these already live in the patient's body anyway, but when your immune system is strong, these germs do not make you sick. There is always a probability that after the transplant, they can cause an infection.

The good news is that most of these infections are easy to treat with antibiotics (NCI, 2022). Two weeks after your transplant, the immune cells will begin recovering. A patient has the highest risk of infection in the first few weeks after the transplant. However, your immune system may need a long time to recover after a transplant. You may need medications to fight infection for about a year or more. Your doctor or healthcare team will talk to you about ways to reduce the risk of infections by taking precautions during your recovery.

Low Blood Cell Count

There is a probability of having a low blood cell count (anemia) after a transplant. Normally, your healthcare team will check your red blood cell count every day. If the count gets too low, you might feel tired, lack energy, and sometimes be breathless. You might need a blood transfusion to top up your red blood cells. This will make you feel better almost right away. Sometimes, people might have allergic reactions to blood transfusions. It is important to inform your healthcare team immediately if you feel hot, shivery, or itchy. They will normally give you medication to stop the reaction. There is a probability that they might slow the transfusion rate. More rarely, some people might have chest or kidney pain, flushed face, chills, and burning around the vein that the drip goes to (NCI, 2022). Again, tell your doctor or nurse immediately if you start having any of the above side effects. They might either stop the reaction or stop the infusion.

Risk of Bleeding

The patient's platelet level will fall after treatment. Platelets help the blood clot. A low platelet count, on the other hand, means you are at risk of bleeding. You might find you are bruising more easily than normal. Patients will experience the following symptoms, which, of course, should be reported immediately. They include nose bleeding, bleeding gums when you clean your teeth, heavy periods for women, blood in the urine, and bruises or small dark red spots on your skin. To help alleviate this situation, your team will arrange for you to have a platelet transfusion, which is normally given in a drip into your vein, and it will take about half an hour. It is not unusual for people to have a reaction to platelets. It will be uncomfortable, but again, inform your nurse or doctor of how you feel. It usually takes longer if you have your own stem cells than if you have donor cells.

Sickness and Diarrhea

Sickness and diarrhea are other side effects associated with bone marrow transplants. You might feel sick after your chemotherapy or radiation therapy. On the other hand, you should start feeling better after a couple of weeks. Sometimes, other treatments you might be having, such as antibiotics, can make you feel weak. Anti-sickness medicine is usually taken as long as you need it (NCI, 2022). Diarrhea is a very common reaction to chemotherapy or radiation therapy. Some people might also have it due to an infection or because they have developed another side effect called graft-versus-host disease.

Sore Mouth

A sore mouth and mouth ulcers are very common after a transplant. They sometimes develop as a reaction to chemotherapy, radiation therapy, or mouth infection. Mouthwash and lozenges to suck can be recommended to help prevent infection. Painkillers and sucking ice cubes can sometimes help to reduce the pain.

Difficulty Eating and Drinking

There is a tendency to lack appetite immediately after transplant. Patients are advised to try small meals throughout the day and whenever they feel like eating. Normally, your dietitian will give you a high-calorie drink if you can't eat much. On the other hand, the patient might have liquid through a tube in the stomach or a central line.

Run Down and Feeling Tired

Patients will feel run down and very tired after their transplant. This will be mostly felt during the second and third weeks when the patient's blood cell counts are at their lowest. Usually, a patient will slowly start having some energy. It is not unusual for a patient to feel more tired than usual for quite a long time after their transplant.

Loss of Fertility

Infertility or loss of fertility is a long-term side effect of a transplant. This, therefore, implies that a patient will no longer be able to get pregnant or father a child naturally. This could be caused by either total body radiation or high doses of chemotherapy. In rare cases, some people who have had transplants do have children naturally, but this is very unusual (NCI, 2022). Young men and teenage boys are usually advised to store their sperm before they start their chemotherapy or radiation. This process is known as sperm banking.

For women, this form of treatment can cause early menopause. To help with the symptoms, women may have hormone replacement therapy. Some women can store embryos or eggs before they start cancer treatment. There is continued research to help women have children after cancer treatment (NCI, 2022).

Graft-versus-Host Disease (GvHD)

Patients who have had a transplant from either a relative or a matched unrelated donor are at risk of GvHD. This is because the donor stem cells contain immune cells from the donor, which can sometimes attack some of the patient's own cells. Graft-versus-host disease can cause diarrhea, weight loss, sore eyes and mouth, skin rashes, shortness of breath, and yellowing of the eyes and skin or jaundice (NCI, 2022).

Graft-versus-host disease can be severe and even life-threatening in some cases. On the other hand, mild GvHD can be helpful for some patients. It is an immune system reaction that can help kill off any cancer cells left after treatment. It is always necessary to let your treatment team know if you have any signs of GvHD. This is mostly treated with an immunosuppressant to help reduce the reaction.

Rejection

It is not unusual for the recipient's body's immune system to reject the transplant, which, of course, happens to be a foreign marrow, especially if the donors are unrelated. Initially, the marrow appears to function, but it fails along the way. Blood counts sometimes may not return to normal, or if they do, the number of blood cells suddenly drops. In most cases, another transplant is scheduled immediately. The second transplant has a higher rate of success because the ability to fight the donor's cells is decreased with immunity-suppressing medications (NCI, 2022).

Immunization Lost

After a transplant, the probability of you losing immunity to diseases you were vaccinated against as a child is too high. It is always important that all your family members have a flu vaccine and that any children in your close family have their childhood immunizations. Some children sometimes have flu vaccines as nasal sprays. If your immune system is severely weakened, you should avoid children who have had the nasal spray two weeks following their vaccination.

Fertility Problems

Fertility problems are a major concern for patients of childbearing age and younger. Because high doses of radiation and chemotherapy make people sterile, some men who are about to undergo a bone marrow transplant should consider banking their sperm before the treatment. For women, the issue is more complicated. Retrieving eggs requires surgery, which is not generally recommended for female bone marrow transplant candidates. Sometimes, even if a woman successfully stores their eggs, it is questionable if their uterus will be able to support the pregnancy after such aggressive cancer treatment. It is noted that women under 25 years of age, however, often maintain their fertility if they do not receive high doses of radiation to their pelvis (NCI, 2022). While bone marrow transplants may not be a major concern for children in the short term, they can potentially delay or halt the onset of puberty.

Learning Problems

It is becoming a common practice to test for learning disabilities as soon as feasible for children who have undergone a bone marrow transplant. Experts have noticed a tendency among children to develop learning disabilities, especially if they have received high doses of radiation to the brain or taken high doses of some chemotherapy drugs (NCI, 2022).

Bone Marrow Transplant and Recurrence

One of the main reasons for bone marrow transplant is the recurrence of the original cancer. New cancers at other sites can also occur after bone marrow transplant. According to the International Bone Marrow Transplant Registry, of some 9,700 bone marrow transplant recipients, about 100 developed a new malignancy during the five to 10 years of follow-up (NCI, 2022).

Some experts believe that treatments designed to destroy the original cancers, such as radiation therapy, chemotherapy, and immune suppression, may predispose a person to develop another cancer (NCI, 2022). To put this risk in perspective, remember that the above modes of treatment were often the only hope for eradicating the original cancer.

Other Complications as a Result of Bone Marrow Transplant

A bone marrow transplant can also cause the following complications: skin rash, cataracts, muscle spasms or leg cramps, numbness in your arms or legs, painful inflammation in your mouth and digestive tract, sleeping problems, blurred vision, stiff joints, and dizzy spells.

Nutritional Facts after Bone Marrow Transplant

Nutritional monitoring and counseling are vital before, during, and after bone marrow transplant. This is because of appetite loss, nausea, vomiting, and other side effects due to the aggressive treatment. To consider individual side effects or differences, experts offer the following advice.

Sometimes, changes in the way food tastes are widespread and may last as long as a couple of months after the bone marrow transplant. The most interesting part of it is the fact that smell perception isn't affected. So, foods with an attractive aroma may stimulate a patient's appetite. If there is no inflammation in your mouth, strong-flavored foods are the most appealing. Patients are advised to avoid bland, unsalted, and overcooked foods. Taste perception eventually returns to normal. Sweet tastes are noted to come back first, followed by bitter, sour, and salty (NCI, 2022).

Dry mouth can make it difficult to chew and swallow foods such as meat and bread. Gravies, soups, broths, or sauces make these foods easier to swallow. Citric acid from lemonade or sugarless lemon drops helps increase saliva production. Patients are also advised to try eating crackers, plain meat, and bananas (NCI, 2022).

Since nausea and vomiting can make eating difficult, try clear liquids, salty foods, and fruits such as watermelon. Avoid very sweet, greasy, and oily foods. Always try eating and drinking slowly while avoiding sudden movements that can precipitate vomiting.

Intravenous feeding may be necessary to ensure an adequate intake of fluids and nutrients. Meal replacement products are not well tolerated immediately after bone marrow transplants. But within a few weeks, such supplements may be helpful. Patients are always advised to work with a dietitian to ensure an adequate intake of food and liquids.

Coping With the Treatment

Studies have shown that after bone marrow transplant, many of the recipients who are placed in laminar airflow rooms feel isolated. Due to the calmness of the room, which is sterile, patients realize, in most cases for the first time, the seriousness of their condition and the demands of their treatment (NCI, 2022).

The feeling of isolation can sometimes be extremely stressful for even the least emotional person. But the combination of isolation and physical discomfort is sometimes particularly distressing. Most bone marrow transplant centers have a social worker available to help the patient, their family, and friends cope during the hospital stay. In some cases, additionally, the center's staff members are trained to deal with the unique issues arising from bone marrow transplants.

According to studies, though a few bone marrow recipients sail through with few psychological repercussions, many become depressed and anxious. Some experts believe that being informed beforehand about the entire process and what emotional stress to expect will help the patient cope better. This will make the patient unfazed by their physical and emotional reactions, and they will be able to accept feelings that otherwise can be construed as abnormal.

Quality of Life

It is noted that the side effects of bone marrow transplant can be very serious for some patients. So, these difficulties raise questions about the quality of life after the transplant. It is especially important for individuals contemplating the procedure to be aware that their life may not return to normal following the recovery from the actual procedure. Poor appetite, vomiting, nausea, and changes in taste may also be some side effects, including skin itching and rashes that even makeup cannot conceal.

Studies show that not everyone has all these experiences, and many bone marrow recipients do return to normal activities. In some surveys, more than 90 percent of the recipients for whom a bone marrow transplant was successful said they could perform normal activities within six months. About eighty percent said their social activities were not impaired or slightly affected, including sex. Severe or even moderate pain was uncommon. More than sixty percent had returned to full-time or part-time work (NCI, 2022).

To improve the outlook, researchers are paying more attention to clarifying areas of unresolved psychological needs. This will, therefore, enable social workers and other healthcare professionals to concentrate on improving the overall quality of life for more people who choose this life-saving procedure.

Bone Marrow Transplant Recovery

The recovery process is different for everyone, but studies show that patients will probably spend several weeks in the hospital. Normally, the patient's immune system will be weak, so they will be taking medications to prevent infections. Sometimes, patients will need a blood transfusion. For the first few weeks, the patient's blood will be checked for engraftment. This might include a sample of the patient's bone marrow (NCI, 2022).

Patients usually leave the hospital after meeting certain criteria, including specific blood cell counts and no fever for two days. Doctors or healthcare workers recommend that before leaving the hospital, a patient should have someone at home to help take care of them. It is also noted that a patient's immune system can take about a year or longer to recover after the transplant. It is recommended that a patient see their doctor often and keep taking medications to prevent infections and graft-versus-host disease, a situation when the new cells attack a patient's own cells.

The patient's medical team may recommend that the patient see a dietitian, who will create a diet plan that will help prevent infection and keep the patient healthy. Other recommendations to the patients will include the avoidance of foods and drinks that carry a high risk of foodborne illnesses. Patients are also asked to choose foods that give their bodies the nutrients they need (See nutrition facts after bone marrow transplant earlier in the chapter).

CHAPTER 18
Cancer Recurrence

Cancer found after cancer treatment and after a period during which cancer couldn't be detected is called cancer recurrence. Sometimes, the current cancer might come back to its original area where it first started or somewhere else in the body. When cancer spreads to new parts of the body, it is named after the part of the body where it first started. An example of such is breast cancer, which might come back in the lymph nodes of the same breast, or it might come back in the other breast or the lungs. On the other hand, it is possible to have cancer later in life after receiving treatment for the initial cancer, which is a separate primary or which is not related to the first one. The fact that a patient was treated, for example, for breast cancer and somewhere along their life develops cervical cancer does not mean they are related.

Normally, a test will be conducted to find out whether it is a new form of cancer that has developed or it is a recurrence of the original cancer. Studies show that it is not possible to predict if cancer is likely to recur after treatment or not (ACS, 2019). On the other hand, the cancer may come back if it is harder to treat because it is fast-growing and or is more advanced and widespread.

Types of Recurrence

Recurrences are labeled based on the distance from the original cancers. There is a **local recurrence,** which means that the cancer has come back to its original location where it started. For instance, a lung that has been treated for cancer is being affected by the same type of cancer.

Secondly, there is a **regional recurrence**. Regional recurrence is a situation where the cancer comes back in the lymph nodes near the place it first started. The chances of this occurring, though minimally, but not ruled out next to the tumor bed, are possible, especially after surgery. Colon cancer is sometimes a good example.

Distance recurrence or metastasis occurs when cancer returns, this time to a different part of the body. Examples of such cases are bone, lung, brain, and liver cancers. Again, most of these cancers can be primary, too.

Some Cancer and Recurrence Description

Controlled

Most often, oncologists might use the term controlled. This is a term used if the test or scans show that the cancer is still in its primary location and is not changing over time. In a nutshell, the tumor or cancer does not appear to be growing. Some tumors are noted to stay the same for a very long time, even without treatment. It is not unusual either for some cancers not to grow after they have been treated, but they must be observed to make sure they are not growing again.

Progressed Cancer

Progressed cancers are cancers that grow or the status of the cancer changes. This growth is relatively based on the providers or the oncologist. Clinical trials look at progressive cancers if they change in size by about 25% from the original (NCI, 2022). It is necessary to inquire with your doctor whenever they use the term because they may be referring to another type of growth.

Sometimes it is hard to differentiate between recurrence and progressive cancers. For example, if cancer has gone for about three months before it comes back, one is not very sure whether it has really gone or not. Chances are that it is not a recurrence of cancer, but more likely that a couple of things might have happened.

First, there is a probability that the surgery done to take out the cancer didn't get all of it. It might be that tiny clusters of cancer cells that couldn't be seen or found on other tests or scans were left behind. They tend to grow large enough over time to show up on scans or cause symptoms. According to studies, these cancers are very aggressive, for they are fast growing and spreading quickly (NCI, 2022).

Secondly, this cancer has become resistant to treatment. Cancer cells are also noted to become resistant to treatment like germs to medication or antibiotics. There is a probability that chemotherapy or radiation therapy might have killed most of the cancer cells, but some were not affected enough by the treatment, and they survived. These cells will grow over time, and they show up as cancer.

According to studies, the shorter the time between when the cancer was thought to have gone and the time it came back, the more aggressive it is. In a nutshell, the more serious the situation. Again, there is no standard length of time to decide if it's recurrence or progression. Most healthcare providers consider recurrence to be cancer that comes back after a patient has no signs of the disease for at least a year (NCI, 2022).

Response and Remission

When cancer is treated and the treatment completely gets rid of the tumor that was seen on tests, scans, or measured in one way or the other, it is known as a complete response or complete remission. A complete response or complete remission does not necessarily mean that the cancer has been cured but that it can no longer be seen on the tests or scans.

Sometimes, there is a partial response or partial remission after treatment. This means that the cancer has been treated and responded to the treatment but has not completely gone away. Partial responses, in most cases, are defined as at least a 50% reduction in tumor measures. The reduction in tumor size must last for at least a month to qualify as a response (NCI, 2022).

Second Cancer

Sometimes, patients make statements such as, "My cancer has come back." While listening to them, you realize that it is a second cancer and not a recurrence. This can be determined after tests or scans are conducted and the results show a new area of cancer and different from the first type. This will, therefore, imply that this individual has a different type of cancer or two primary cancers. These two types of cancers might have started from two types of cells under microscopic examination. Having two types of cancer is rare, but it does happen (ACS, 2019).

Note that having cancer once does not mean that you can't get another form of cancer in the future. The fact that a patient has a second type of cancer independent of the first means that these two forms of cancer will be approached differently as far as treatment is concerned (NCI, 2022).

CHAPTER 19
Combination Treatments

Over the years, it is not unusual for cancer to be treated by more than one method of treatment because it has proven to be more effective. A combination of surgery, chemotherapy, and radiation therapy may be more effective than a single therapy alone. Studies have shown that under certain conditions, combination treatment can achieve a greater likelihood of cure than a single mode of treatment with even less damage to vital tissues and organs (NCI, 2022).

Huge successes, among others, are noted in the use of combination therapies for the treatment of osteosarcoma, a bone cancer found mostly in young people (Murphy, G.P., Morris, L.B., & Lange, D., 1997). Compared to years ago, when amputation of the affected limb was the only method of treatment, radiation is directed to the affected area, and chemotherapy is directed through the bloodstream, treating the cancer without losing the limb with cancer. Treatment of breast cancer happens to be another good example of the success of combination treatment. Previous forms of treatment entailed the removal of the whole breast, or mastectomy, which is outdated, especially in the Western world. Recent and better forms of treatment for breast cancer include lumpectomy, which is the excision of the lump followed by radiation therapy. This allows women to retain their breast shape without compromising the treatment. The treatment of small cell lung cancer with the use of chemotherapy and radiation therapy, which in most cases gives good results, is another area of success for combination therapy (ACS, 2019).

Reasons for Combined Cancer Treatment

Studies have shown that multidimensional approaches to the treatment of cancer have proven to be more successful than a single mode of treatment. That is why sometimes doctors combine two or three standard treatments, in some cases, experimental therapies, to treat certain types of cancer (NCI, 2022).

The reasons for this type of treatment vary from patient to patient, but in most cases, oncologists take into consideration some of the following factors. It is noted that one form of treatment may enhance the effectiveness of another. Sometimes, the side effects to the patient might be such that you may want to discontinue the treatment, but using two or more methods of treatment may reduce the extent or intensity of another. It is also possible that a single approach alone may not affect the tumor.

Now, multidimensional therapy requires a well-planned strategy designed to exploit the unique qualities of each of the component treatments. The strengths and weaknesses of all the combined treatments should be balanced, thereby increasing the level of success. To recommend this approach, healthcare providers take into consideration the type of cancer, the size of the tumor, and how fast the cancer spreads either locally or to other organs (NCI, 2022). Depending on the stage, the doctor chooses the approach which might have the greatest impact on the cancer. This approach to treatment is recommended in most cases with the possibility of curing the cancer. In this case, the secondary treatments may come either after, before, or at the same time as the primary type.

In most cases, the approaches are equally weighted. Thus, it is difficult to distinguish which of the approaches is primary and which is secondary. Certain cancers, such as breasts, are a good example of a multidimensional approach to treatment, which might include surgery, chemotherapy, and radiation therapy. Failure to apply either one or two of the treatment types may lead to poor results.

The mixture and sequence of the therapies and sometimes surgery depends chiefly on the risk of the spread and speed at which the cancer cells divide. Rapidly or slowly dividing cells, alongside factors such as the age of the patient, general health, and the ability to tolerate the therapy, must be taken into consideration. The fact that various modalities may interact in ways that vary with the type and stage of the cancers, patients should always bear in mind that though two people may all have the same type of cancer, say breast, the approach to tackling it might be different.

It is very important that the physician discusses the treatment plan with the patient, including other options, in advance of their action. Sometimes, some changes may be made, especially if a patient is having either a very positive response to a drug or an advent or negative reaction to a certain medication. Your doctor will then study the situation carefully before coming up with another game plan. In such a situation, the doctor will have a proper discussion with you and your family to notify you why the change of actions, and it is important for you and your family to ask questions to clear up every doubt or concern you might have.

Usually, combination therapy requires a team approach, using the expertise of several doctors to ensure the most effective approach and timing with the most benefit to the patient and with the least risk. For example, your primary doctor, pathologist, oncologist, surgeon, and other providers draw up a plan that is suitable for your individual case. What they will be discussing among themselves is how to prioritize the treatment options to minimize conflicts. In some situations, radiation therapy might be the primary mode of treatment to help shrink a tumor before surgery. In other instances, surgery is first performed, and later radiation therapy. What the team might take into consideration are the effects of the treatment method on the surrounding tissues and organs, and if it will affect the healing process.

Normally, the team agrees on the treatment plan before the implementation. That is why the patient and their family must choose a good primary care doctor who will help coordinate this plan. Sometimes, it is important to select a family member, friend, or nurse navigator who will be doing this coordination, which might be very overwhelming.

Neoadjuvant Therapy

Surgery, for a long time, has been the first treatment of choice for many doctors when they have to recommend treatment for their patients with cancer. However, with the advancement in cancer care, this is not always the case anymore. Nowadays, surgery is not always the primary sequence of treatment. The sequence is based on the type of cancer, stage, and treatment circumstances.

In a situation where cancer has spread to other areas, the doctor might order radiation therapy, chemotherapy, or both before surgery to reduce the size of the tumor, thus making it suitable for surgery, which at this moment will be less drastic.

Chemotherapy

Studies show that chemotherapy before radiation therapy or surgery is not a very popular sequence of cancer treatment (NCI, 2022). But sometimes, it is very useful in shrinking the size of the cancer, thus enabling a less dramatic type of surgery. Chemotherapy is often also recommended if the cancer is very aggressive and might not respond to other methods of treatment as well.

Radiation Therapy

Sometimes, doctors are concerned about cancer cells dislodging during surgery and spreading elsewhere in the body. To avoid this, they prescribe neoadjuvant radiation therapy. It is not unusual for cancer cells to linger around the tumor bed as well. Radiation therapy will help reduce the likelihood of these cells multiplying or spreading. It will also help shrink the size of the tumor, thus making it suitable for a comfortable and successful surgery.

Treatment Schedules

Normally, treatment schedules vary depending on a couple of things, which include the type of cancer, the extent of spread, and the physical condition of the patient. When doctors are timing any neoadjuvant therapy, they take into consideration how each treatment type works and how it relates to the other types of treatments. Sometimes, radiation therapy is the first mode of treatment before surgery. There may be a couple of hours or days in between. Chemotherapy, on the other hand, may be administered to a patient a couple of months before radiation therapy, especially for head and neck cancers.

Radiation therapy as a neoadjuvant treatment is usually given in doses over a short period to kill and destroy cancer cells, minimize the side effects to the patient, and incur the least delay possible before surgery. Though there is a lot of improvement in the radiation therapy modes of treatment, this treatment usually takes a week to two, followed by two weeks of recovery before surgery.

Risks and complications

Studies show that all cancer therapies have some side effects and can sometimes cause complications, but combining them doesn't necessarily mean that there is a probability of greater risk (ACS, 2019). On the other hand, when a therapy poses a risk, the doctor chooses it only if the benefits outweigh the complications that may arise from the side effects.

It is noted that if chemotherapy and radiation therapy are given first in the treatment plan, there is a likelihood of some potential side effects of surgery. Some of these complications include but are not limited to adhesions of tissues, fistulas, fibrosis, and abscesses (ACS, 2019). Radiation therapy may also trigger side effects from subsequent chemotherapy. Certain chemotherapy drugs given after radiation therapy may trigger sunburn-like reactions in the more sensitive skin in the area treated with radiation. Patients undergoing this form of treatment are always advised not to spend much time in the sun.

Again, the risks of combination therapy may be high because of the side effects. All the possibilities should be part of the treatment planning decision. Experienced doctors carefully monitor during treatment. They use the safest and most effective doses and continuous teamwork is very necessary to prevent or manage most side effects and complications.

Advantages

Though there might be some amount of risks involved in neoadjuvant therapy, there are advantages to this approach. Studies show that people are stronger and in a better nutritional state and may tolerate radiation therapy or chemotherapy before surgery (ACS, 2019).

Secondly, since the blood supply has not yet been interrupted by surgery, chemotherapy can reach the tumor in high concentration. It is also noted that a good oxygen supply through the bloodstream also makes the cancer cells more susceptible to radiation, studies show (ACS, 2019).

Neoadjuvant therapy is noted to provide a guide for treatment. This is because a good response to chemotherapy before surgery usually indicates a good or similar response to chemotherapy after surgery. This mode of treatment is also noted to be advantageous because large numbers of growing cells can be destroyed.

Adjuvant Therapy

Adjuvant therapy is a combined treatment that has a sequence, with surgery being the first type of treatment to be administered. The tumor is taken out by surgery and later treated by either radiation therapy or chemotherapy, or both. To recommend this mode of treatment means that the cancer is still localized (ACS, 2019). This supplemental local treatment of radiation therapy kills any cancer cells remaining in the immediate area or treatment of chemotherapy that can destroy cancer cells in other parts of the body. Your doctor will take into consideration the type of cancer, whether there is a danger of recurrence, whether the cancer is still localized or not, and the spread or growth of the cancer cells.

Treatment Timing

Usually, chemotherapy begins as soon as possible after surgery after allowing little time for recovery from the surgery. Radiation therapy after surgery must be delayed till after the wound has healed. It is not unusual for chemotherapy to be administered after radiation therapy. Studies show that the longer the delay of chemotherapy, the lower the chances of cure (ACS, 2019).

Advantages

Studies show that performing surgery first allows the surgeon, pathologist, oncologist, and radiologist to review the result of the surgery, which is examining the size and the type of tumor that was removed and the cells from the surrounding area. This analysis by the team helps to determine if post-radiation therapy will be necessary or not. It will make the cost less expensive to the patient, especially after examination, and they conclude that radiation will not be beneficial to the patient.

Having surgery first, on the other hand, might be disadvantageous in the sense that it may reduce the oxygen supply to tumor cells, making them resistant to radiation therapy. Performing surgery first, in some cases, is especially noted to be disadvantageous in situations like abdominal surgery, which might make other parts of the body, like the small intestine, susceptible to damage from radiation therapy if they must administer it (ACS, 2019).

Observations

Studies show that adjunctive radiation therapy and chemotherapy may have the same side effects as though either of the two was administered separately. Still, on the other hand, studies equally show that they don't have additional side effects if the two are combined or will aggravate the effects. This will be true, especially if the patient is given enough time to recover from the surgery. It is also noted that long-term effects from the surgery don't seem to change the side effects of radiation therapy or chemotherapy (ACS, 2019).

Chemotherapy and Radiation Therapy

The approach of radiation therapy and chemotherapy combination is commonly used when there is a known likelihood of recurrence or when there is evidence of cancer spreading to another area. The oncologist will use this combination of radiation therapy and chemotherapy to treat both the primary and the distant disease. Now, there are certain situations whereby a combination of radiation therapy and chemotherapy is used without surgery, especially if the cancer is not still localized.

The application of radiation therapy and chemotherapy to treat certain cancers is very advantageous. This is because each attacks the volume of cells differently, especially when it comes to large tumor masses versus microscopic, scattered cells. It is noted that chemotherapy given first can shrink the tumor while making it more susceptible to radiation therapy, which works best on small tumors (ACS, 2019).

It is also worthwhile noting that the effects of chemotherapy and radiation therapy are supplementary to each other depending on the cancer cells' rate of growth. While radiation therapy works better against older and slow-growing cells, chemotherapy is good for the young and the more aggressive ones (ACS, 2019).

The use of both therapies in some cases makes the other possible. For some cancers like the head and neck, chemotherapy may be given a few months before radiation therapy begins. Sometimes, chemotherapy may be administered simultaneously with radiation therapy to make the cells more vulnerable to radiation. Rectal cancer is one of those cancers where a combination of radiation therapy and chemotherapy gives a better result compared to the sum of one of each (ACS, 2019).

Intraoperative Radiation Therapy

Intraoperative radiation is a situation in which radiation is used to treat cancer during an operation. After the tumor has been exposed or removed, the oncologist uses high doses of radiation directed to the tumor site before the wound is closed. This is usually a single fraction of radiation that is precisely targeted while sparing the surrounding normal tissues, skin, or organs, which are shielded with lead to prevent them from exposure. Sometimes, intraoperative radiation is given in addition to postoperative radiation therapy. Depending on the facility, this process could either be undertaken in a radiation oncology department or the operating room. Some of the most suitable cancers for intraoperative radiation therapy include pancreatic, breast, colon, and female reproductive organs (ACS, 2019).

Immunotherapy and Surgery

The combination of surgery and immunotherapy is known to help shrink the tumor as well as prompt a patient's body to release attacker cells to reach smaller tumors. It is noted that patients who receive immunotherapy before and after surgery live almost twice as long as those who only receive immunotherapy once before the surgery (ACS, 2019). Though research is still ongoing, studies show that immunotherapy before surgery may greatly shrink certain tumors, especially those of the colon and oral (ACS, 2019).

Immunotherapy with Chemotherapy

The treatment of cancer with a combination of chemotherapy and immunotherapy is also becoming popular. Sometimes, cancer spreads to lymph nodes, and it may return after radiation therapy and chemotherapy. Researchers have found that chemotherapy and immunotherapy are helpful and safe. The combination of chemotherapy and immunotherapy is noted to be very beneficial in the treatment of pancreatic, lung, blood, leukemia, and cervical cancers (ACS, 2019).

When chemotherapy is used along with immunotherapy, the benefits are noted to go beyond using the combination of drugs. Again, immunotherapy drugs work by helping the immune system recognize and attack cancer cells. When cancer cells are broken down by chemotherapy drugs, it can help the immune system recognize these cells as abnormal so that the immunotherapy drugs can be more effective.

Lifestyle and Nutrition Advice

It should be noted that while receiving combination therapy to treat cancer, the body needs support from our diet, immune system, and overall health. Alcohol should be avoided. This is because it does not only cause cancer but is also linked to a range of possible effects on the risks posed by cancer to those recently diagnosed.

The patient is advised to try to ensure the intake of the recommended daily number of vitamins and minerals each day through their diet. This helps to build cells, keeping them healthy while repairing damage and preventing further complications. A healthy diet that includes plenty of variety and lots of antioxidant fruits and vegetables is recommended. Intake of high-fiber grains like beans and whole grains may help reduce the risk of a second cancer (ACS, 2019).

It is necessary that the patient does the recommended daily amount of exercise and to try maintaining a daily regular exercise regime as much as they can. On the other hand, if you are not up to the exercise after the treatment, allow the body to rest and fully recover to later return to the recommended routine. Again, consult with your healthcare team for guidance.

Questions for your Doctor

1. What are the side effects of this type of treatment? If there are any, are they going to be permanent?

2. Do you have any track records to prove that this type of treatment works very well for my type of cancer?

3. Who are the members of my treatment team and is there going to be a member of this team who will be doing the coordination?

4. Is there a possibility of skipping the next step of the treatment if my cancer proves responsive after the first treatment?

5. Are the side effects from the first treatment going to delay the next? For instance, if the effects from my first mode of treatment, either chemotherapy or radiation therapy, are terrible, is this going to delay the surgery?

6. What are the consequences if I choose to discontinue the treatment?

7. How long is my treatment going to take? How long will I be in the hospital, and will I be able to work and travel after my treatment?

8. Will I lose my hair and how long is it going to take to grow back to its original state?

9. Will this treatment interfere with my sexuality?

10. What is the cost of this treatment and is my insurance going to cover the whole cost?

11. Is there a clinical trial for my type of cancer, and if there is one, who do I talk to, and what might be the qualifications to be able to participate?

12. From your experience, how long is it going to take for me to recover?

CHAPTER 20
Other Developments

Studies show that cancer specialists are constantly seeking new and improved methods of treating cancer. As improved methods are coming up after research, so too do they adjust. Investigative ways to improve this is through clinical research trials. Some of the ways this is conducted are by the addition of biological therapy, drugs that boost the body's natural immune defense (NCI, 2022).

Hormones or hormone suppressants are also being added to enhance chemotherapy in some treatment plans for cancers that are influenced by the hormonal environment, such as the cancers of the prostate, breast, uterus, and thyroid. Bone marrow transplants include other methods that are increasingly used, whereby vital stem cells that were destroyed by chemotherapy are restored (NCI, 2022).

Footnotes

Sometimes, people are irregular with their medical appointments or stop their cancer treatment. It is not unusual for people undergoing combination treatment to be noncompliant because the treatments are long-term, expensive, and sometimes inconvenient. The reasons for this inconvenience could be transportation difficulties to and from the doctor's office, out-of-pocket expenses, and depression from the fact that they have such an illness. "Why me" is a popular question from a lot of patients.

Some patients respond dramatically to the first part of the treatment plan, and they think they are cured and don't need to proceed with therapy, especially if they expect some serious side effects from the next mode of treatment. It should be noted that multi-approach is an overall strategy that, to be successful, needs to be completed. Again, it is in the interest of the patient to have a full course of their treatment. If there are any concerns at any point, your healthcare team is ready to provide the necessary assistance you might require. Do not hesitate to ask questions or have your concerns addressed.

Hormone Therapy

Hormone therapy, also known as hormonal therapy, hormone treatment, or endocrine therapy, is a type of cancer treatment that slows or stops the growth of cancer that uses hormones to grow. To treat cancer, hormone therapy is effective in preventing and the reduction of symptoms in men with prostate cancer who are not able to have radiation therapy or surgery (ACS, 2019).

Hormone therapy falls into two groups: those that block the body's ability to produce hormones and those that interfere with how hormones behave in the body. Prostate and breast cancers that use hormones to grow are two types of cancers that are known to be treated using hormone therapy (ACS, 2019). Hormone therapy is most often used along with other cancer treatments. The types of treatment that a patient needs depend on the type of cancer, whether it has spread or not and how far, if the growth involves hormones, and if the patient has other health issues.

Benefits of Hormone Therapy

Hormone therapy, when used with other forms of cancer treatment, makes a tumor smaller before surgery or radiation therapy as a form of neoadjuvant therapy. As an adjuvant therapy, it lowers the risk of a recurrence after the main treatment. Hormone therapy is also known to destroy cancer cells that have returned or spread to other parts of the body (NCI, 2022).

Side Effects

Unwanted side effects may occur from hormone therapy. This is because hormone therapy blocks the body's ability to produce hormones and sometimes interferes with hormone behaviors. The side effects depend on the type of hormone therapy that an individual receives and how their body responds to it. Studies show that people might respond differently to the same treatment. This, therefore, means that not every patient has the same side effects. Sometimes, side effects differ between the genders.

For men, some common side effects include hot flashes, diarrhea, nausea, loss of interest or the ability to have sex, weakened bones, fatigue, and enlarged breasts. Women will have some of the above side effects, including changes in their mood, vaginal dryness, and changes in their periods if they have not yet reached menopause (NCI, 2022).

How Hormone Therapy is Given

Hormone therapy is administered to patients in a couple of ways. One of the channels in which hormone therapy is administered is oral; this is when pills are swallowed. Hormone therapy can also be administered through injections, which are typically given into a muscle such as the arm, thigh, or hip or just beneath the skin in the fatty areas of the abdomen or leg. Sometimes, a patient may have surgery to remove organs that produce hormones. In men, the testicles are removed, while in women, it is their ovaries which are removed.

Now, where a patient receives treatment depends on which hormone therapy they are getting and how it is given. The most likely environment to take hormone therapy is either at home, a doctor's clinic, or the hospital.

Biomarker Testing for Cancer Treatment

This is a way of testing to look for genes, proteins, and other substances called biomarkers or tumor markers that can provide information about cancer. Each patient's cancer has a unique pattern of biomarkers. Some of these biomarkers affect how certain cancer treatment works. Biomarker testing is a useful tool for the patient and their doctor's choice of treatment for their type of cancer. This is most useful for people with solid and blood cancers (NCI, 2022). Biomarker testing is equally known to help doctors diagnose and monitor cancers during and after treatment.

Uses of Biomarkers Test to Select Cancer Treatment

Biomarkers are an important tool for helping patients and their doctors select cancer treatments. Some treatments, such as targeted therapy and immunotherapy, may only work for patients whose cancers have certain biomarkers (NCI, 2022).

Biomarkers also make it possible to treat patients with certain genetic changes. In this case, biomarker testing can determine whether someone's cancer has a gene change that can be treated with an inhibitor.

Biomarker testing can also help patients find a new study of cancer treatment, which might be a clinical trial that could be helpful in treating your form of cancer. It is not unusual for some studies to enroll people based on the biomarkers in their cancers instead of the part of the body where the cancer started growing. These are ongoing research, which is sometimes basket trials (NCI, 2022).

Biomarkers as Part of Precision Medicine

Biomarkers are part of precision medicine, also known as personalized medicine. Precision medicine is an approach to medical care in which disease prevention, diagnosis, and treatment are tailored to the genes, proteins, and other substances of a patient's body. For cancer treatment, precision medicine means using biomarkers and other tests to select treatments that are likely to help a patient (NCI, 2022). By the same token, it helps to spare the patient from treatments that are not likely to be helpful to them.

Precision medicine is not a new idea, but recent advances in science and technology are helping to speed up the pace in this area of research. Though more is still to be discovered, scientists now understand that cancer cells have many different changes in genes, proteins, and other substances that make the cells grow and spread. Scientists have also learned that though two people may have the same type of cancer, they may likely have different changes in their cancers. It is worthwhile noting that some of these changes affect how certain cancer treatments work (NCI, 2022).

It is important to note that even though researchers are making progress daily, the precision medicine approach to cancer treatment is not yet part of routine care for most cancer cases. Conversely, it is also important to note that even the standard approach to cancer treatment, which is selected based on the type of cancer, size, and where it has spread, is effective and personalized to each patient (NCI, 2022).

Ways of Conducting Biomarker Testing

After considering all the options a patient may have and having decided with their healthcare team on biomarker testing as part of their care, they will take a sample of their cancer cells. Normally, if a patient is having surgery for solid tumors, they will take a sample of the cells during surgery. On the other hand, if the patient is not having surgery, they may need to have a biopsy of the tumor.

For patients who have blood cancer or are getting a biomarker test done, known as liquid biopsy, the patient will need to have their blood drawn. A patient might have a liquid biopsy test done, especially if their tumor is hard to reach with a needle.

The patient's sample will be sent to a special lab where it will be tested for biomarkers. The lab will then create a report that lists the biomarkers in the cancer cells and whether any treatments might work. The patient's healthcare team will discuss the results and eventually decide on a treatment (NCI, 2022).

For biomarker tests that analyze genes, a patient will need to give their healthy cells. This is usually done by collecting a patient's blood, saliva, or a small piece of skin. These tests compare the patient's cancer cells with their healthy cells to find genetic changes that arose during a patient's lifetime.

Types of Biomarker Tests

Many types of biomarker tests can help select a cancer treatment. Most biomarker tests used to select cancer treatment look for genetic markers. On the other hand, some look for proteins or other kinds of markers (NCI, 2022).

Some tests check for a single marker, while others check for many biomarkers at the same time. These are called multi-gene tests or panel tests. The Oncotype DX test is an example of a test that looks at the activity of about 21 different genes to predict whether chemotherapy is likely to work for someone with breast cancer.

Some tests look for biomarkers that are found in many types of cancer and can be used by people with different kinds of cancers. On the other hand, some tests are case-specific for certain cancers like melanoma. Some tests called whole exome sequencing (WES) look at all the genes in your cancer. Others, such as whole genome sequencing, look at all the DNA in your cancer, which includes both genes and outside of genes (NCI, 2022).

Other biomarker tests look at the number of genetic changes in a patient's cancer, known as tumor mutational burden. This information can be helpful in figuring out if a type of immunotherapy known as immune checkpoint inhibitors may work for your form of cancer. Liquid biopsies are other known biomarker tests. These tests look in blood and other fluids for biomarkers from cancer cells. Some examples are Guardant360 CDx and FoundationOne Liquid CDx (NCI, 2022).

The Meaning of a Biomarker Test Result

Like any informative result, a biomarker test could show that your cancer has a certain biomarker that is targeted by a certain therapy. This means that the therapy may work to treat your cancer. Matching therapy may be available as an off-label treatment, through participation in clinical trials, or as an FDA-approved treatment.

In many cases, biomarker testing may find changes in a patient's cancer that will not help the patient's doctor make treatment decisions. This occurs in situations where genetic changes that are thought to be benign, that are harmless, or whose effects are not known or of unknown significance are not used to make treatment decisions (NCI, 2022).

Based on your test results, your oncologist may recommend a treatment that is not yet approved by the FDA for your cancer type. This might be because this treatment has been approved for the treatment of a different type of cancer that has the same biomarker as your cancer. It, therefore, implies that the treatment is used off-label, but it may work for you because your cancer has the biomarker that this treatment targets (ACS, 2019).

Sometimes, biomarker tests could find genetic changes in an individual that they might have been born with, which increases the individual's risk of cancer or other diseases. Such genetic changes are also known as germline mutations. Usually, if such changes are found, the individual may need another genetic test to confirm whether the individual truly has an inherited mutation that increases their cancer risk.

Finding out that an individual has an inherited mutation that increases the risk of cancer may affect this individual and their family. Because of this reason, the healthcare provider may recommend that you talk with either a genetic healthcare provider such as a clinical geneticist, genetic counselor, or a genetic nurse to help you understand what the test results might mean to you and your family.

Sometimes, the result could also show that an individual's cancer has a biomarker that may prevent a certain therapy from working. This information could spare a patient from getting a treatment that will not be helpful for their situation.

Shortcomings

Biomarker tests are known not to help everyone who gets them. There are several reasons why they may not help certain individuals.

One of the reasons biomarker tests may not be helpful is that the biomarkers in a patient's cancer can change over time. A test is known to only capture a snapshot of the changes at one point in time. This, therefore, means that the results of a biomarker test done in the past may not reflect the biomarkers in an individual's cancer now. Your oncologist may want to test your disease again if there is a recurrence or a second cancer (NCI, 2022).

Another reason the treatment might not work is that not all of a patient's cancer cells have the same biomarkers. This means that a biomarker test may find a treatment that can kill some but not all of your cancer cells. The cancer cells that are not killed by the treatment could keep growing, preventing the treatment from working or increasing the chances of recurrence (NCI, 2022).

Research has also shown that even if an individual's test finds a biomarker that matches an available treatment, the therapy may not work for all. Sometimes, other features of a patient's cancer or their body affect how well a treatment works. This may include how an individual's body breaks down the medicine.

Other reasons include the fact that the test identifies a matching therapy that is being tested in a clinical trial in which you are not able to participate. Sometimes, a patient is unable to safely get a biopsy needed for testing. It is not unusual in situations where there is not enough tumor tissue in an individual's biopsy sample to have biomarker testing done. It could be that the test does not find a biomarker in a patient's cancer that matches the available therapies.

CHAPTER 21
Clinical Trials

Treatment of cancer has not been locked down yet. That is why scientific studies involving human beings are crucial to conquering the disease. Investigations have led to a greater understanding of how cancer progresses, the development of more precise methods of diagnosing and detection, and the planning of highly effective prevention and treatment strategies.

Clinical trials are research practices that are designed to follow ethical medical practices with the intent of providing current standards of treatment. In the United States, these standards have been approved and laid down by the College of Oncologists, Scientists, the National Institute of Health (NIH), the FDA, and the American Cancer Society. Most people participate in these trials because new drugs are approved, and a continuous alteration in regimens is made to ensure that the participants receive the up-to-date therapies available.

Normally, the candidates for clinical trials are on a voluntary basis. The potential benefits of volunteering for clinical trials vary depending on the stage of the research. It is noted that in the earlier stages, the benefits are limited. This is because the purpose of these studies is to establish whether the treatment or drug should be evaluated. Conversely, in the last phase, where the prospect of the drug or treatment is good, the potential for benefits is greater. Most people like to enter trials in the last phase because they want to be the first beneficiaries of the new treatment, especially if the new treatment is superior to what is currently on the market (NCI, 2022).

It is noted that some people volunteer knowing that the trial will not help them, but they are satisfied with the fact that they are helping to solve the mystery disease. On the other hand, studies show that less than 5 percent of adults with cancer will want to participate in clinical trials. Still, scientists believe that if more people volunteer, there will be a significant improvement in detection, diagnosis, and treatment. About half of those with cancer are cured, especially in developed countries, but the number could climb considerably if more people volunteer for trials (NCI, 2022). Studies show that there is a progressive accomplishment due to trials on children's cancers such as Wilms' tumor, neuroblastoma, Ewing's sarcoma, and acute lymphocytic leukemia (Murphy, G.P., Morris, L.B., & Lange, D., 1997).

Researchers all over the world are investigating and studying what causes cancer, diagnosing and how to prevent it. Some study after treatments on the patient, and some aim at developing better ways of controlling some of cancer's most devastating effects, like pain. Statistics show that researchers are mostly focused on clinical trials to test and improve potential treatment methods. Some of these include new chemotherapy drugs or different combinations, innovative radiation therapy techniques with chemotherapy and or surgery, and various biological therapies, either alone or in combination with other treatment methods (NCI, 2022).

While researchers are looking for ways to help cure the disease, they often examine how particular treatments may help enhance a patient's quality of life. This is aimed at boosting an individual's morals, reducing psychological stress, and relieving pain and other symptoms while allowing the patient to continue working and enjoying life.

The Importance of Clinical Trials

The importance of clinical trials cannot be overemphasized. People nowadays are living longer because of successful cancer treatments and because of past clinical trials. Studies show that through clinical trials, doctors and scientists determine whether new treatments are safe and effective and work better than the current treatments. Again, these trials help improve quality of life, and when you take part in these trials, you add to an already immense amount of knowledge about cancer and help improve cancer care for future patients. Clinical trials are the key to making progress against cancer. It is very necessary or important that all ethnic groups participate in clinical trials.

Informed Consent Before Clinical Trial

This agreement details the potential benefits and risks that may arise from this clinical trial. It is very important for every person undergoing a clinical trial to understand the risks involved in that trial. Some of these risks are unknown to a greater extent, and the patient must be aware of this by making sure every question or doubt from the patient's side is answered.

The consent form for clinical trials is always lengthy and, in most cases, detailed with a lot of medical terms that an ordinary patient may not understand or be familiar with. It is, therefore, very necessary that your healthcare team or doctor explain to you every detail of what is involved in the clinical trial before signing the form. Sometimes, it is advisable to bring an outside provider or family member who can ask questions on your behalf. In a nutshell, a patient is given the opportunity to fully understand what they are going to put themselves into. That is why some facilities will allow potential candidates for trials to take home the forms to make sure they clearly understand the content before signature.

It is important to note that even though a patient has signed the consent form, they are not legally bound to complete the clinical trial. Though there might be some variations on the consent form between facilities, they must state that you will regularly attend your trials and that you will be updated regarding the trials, including toxicity, if any. On the other hand, if either the patient or their doctor determines that they are experiencing some abnormalities that are not suitable for continuity, the clinical trial can be terminated immediately.

Compassion Situation

There are situations where a drug on trial is promising, and there is a lot of publicity for it, but the trial is not yet complete and approved by the FDA or the approval authority. In this case, an argument can be made as a form of compassionate need, which is a process that has been developed allowing cancer patients who have exhausted all other forms of treatment to receive the experimental drug. Normally, the use of this drug will be called off by the protocol. This, therefore, implies that this patient is not part of a clinical trial, even if they qualify (NCI, 2022).

Phases of Clinical Trials

In most cases, clinical trials on cancer are undertaken by large government agencies like the National Cancer Institute in the United States, the Department of Health in the UK, and big pharmaceutical companies. This is because clinical trials are long, slow, and often very expensive undertakings. Studies show that a clinical trial may take up to 15 years to be conclusive (NCI, 2022).

Prior to human testing of a drug, researchers conduct rigorous preliminary experiments in test tubes and on animals to determine which drug is likely to affect cancer and make an educated guess on how to administer the drug. If laboratory research shows promising results, a government agency such as the FDA in the United States approves the drug for investigation and gives the go-ahead for human studies.

Clinical trials are usually conducted in phases that build upon one another. Each phase answers questions that are mostly designed, and knowing the phase of the clinical trial is important because it gives you an idea of how much is known about the treatment being undertaken. There are risks and benefits to taking part in clinical trials. Again, the benefits outweigh the risks, and it is not much like a guinea pig as such because these trials are conducted under approved standards.

Phase 0

This phase of clinical trials is intended to speed up and streamline the drug approval process. Studies show that Phase 0 studies may help researchers find out if the drugs meet the anticipated expectations. By doing so, time and money that could be spent on later phases are saved if there is no positive predicted outcome.

In this phase, only a few small doses of a new drug are used on a few people. This is to test whether the drug reaches the tumor, how the drug acts in the human body, and how the cancer cells in the human body respond to the drug. As part of the process, people in the study may need extra tests such as biopsies, scans, and blood samples.

This phase of clinical trials, unlike other phases, does not benefit people who participate at this level of the trial. This only benefits other people in the future. On the other hand, since drug doses are low, there are also fewer risks for the patients who are in this trial (NCI, 2022).

Phase 0 studies are noted not to be widely used, and some drugs might not be helpful. Studies at this phase of the clinical trial are usually very small, often with fewer than 20 people, and the drug is given only for a short period (NCI, 2022). This phase is not a required part of the testing process of a new drug. The fact that there is no direct benefit to the people participating in this phase, most volunteers for these studies fall under the good Samaritan category.

Phase I

Phase I studies of a new drug typically mark the first stage of testing in humans. This initial investigation of treatment is to test the safety and effectiveness of a promising new therapy and to learn if it is worthy of further investigation. In the case of a new drug, this is when researchers learn about its effects by gradually increasing the dosage stepwise and carefully analyzing the response among the participants.

Usually, it is in this phase of the clinical trials that researchers find out how well the body absorbs a drug, how much reaches the bloodstream, and how it is metabolized and eliminated from the body. Based on the results obtained, scientists will then decide if a larger study will be possible that will reveal the potential effectiveness of the drug.

Because participants in Phase I of the studies experience toxic and other side effects, the number is usually very small, sometimes about 12 people (NCI, 2022). Usually, a patient will not be considered for this phase of the study unless the patient's cancer is in the advanced stage and other conventional therapies have been employed without success, and this is the last option. In a nutshell, people who enter this phase of the trials have no other treatment possibilities, and this may offer some hope.

Placebos or inactive treatments are not used in Phase I clinical trials, though they carry the most potential risks. In this phase, for those with life-threatening diseases, weighing the potential risks and benefits carefully is key, and some patients choose to join this stage of the trial when every other option has been exhausted.

Phase II

After researchers have found the potential of a new treatment at the completion of Phase I of the clinical trial, Phase II of the trial is now recommended. In Phase II, a drug is tested on how it works on certain types of cancers. In this phase, safe dosages and other specifics of administration are determined. Usually, the number of participants is slightly higher than that in Phase I. What doctors are looking for at this phase is based on their goals, which might be to see how cancer shrinks or to achieve complete disappearance. It might mean long periods when the cancer does not get bigger, or it might mean a long period before there is a recurrence. Some trials may be aimed at improving the quality of life for patients.

Sometimes, clinical trials look to see if patients who get the new treatment live longer than patients who do not have the treatment.

In some ways, this phase of the clinical trial is a preview of a new treatment. It is not unusual for the results not to indicate for certain that the treatment is an improvement on a current form of treatment. It might show the potential to be a better treatment.

During this phase of the trial, participants in this case have been treated with standard treatments before they had a relapse or recurrence of their disease. Doctors recommend this to their patients because, since the cancers have not responded well to the standard therapies, they want to exhaust all the options for the well-being of their patients and the belief that it will be beneficial to them.

Researchers gather information on how patients respond by sometimes measuring the size of the tumor for shrinkage or analyzing blood cell samples in cases of blood cancers like leukemia. Sometimes, the patient's tumor markers are measured, which often indicates whether the cancer is growing or shrinking.

Usually, in Phase II of clinical trials, every patient gets the same dose of the drug. Sometimes, during this phase, patients are randomly assigned to different treatment groups. These groups may get different doses or get the treatment in different ways to justify which provides the best balance of response and safety. Placebos or inactive treatments are not used in this phase. If fewer side effects are seen and more patients benefit from this phase, Phase III of the clinical trial begins.

Phase III

Phase III is the final phase of the clinical trial. Usually, treatments that have been proven to work in Phase II of the trial must succeed in the final phase to be approved for standard consumption or treatment (NCI, 2022). At this phase of the clinical trial, the effectiveness of the new drug or treatment is compared to the available standard.

Participants at this stage of the clinical trial typically have the same type and stage of cancer, and they usually number in the hundreds, often across multiple facilities and, when possible, in various locations around the world. This is because the level of improvement may be small, and many subjects in different locations are needed to determine reliable statistical methods if the benefits are better than the standard treatments.

This phase of the clinical trial is designed to help doctors determine if the new treatment is better, inferior, or equal to the standard treatments. Participants at this stage are supposed to be receiving this treatment and this treatment alone and have not received any other treatment for their disease. This will enable scientists to know that any change in the participants' conditions is due to the treatment they receive in the study and not from any other form of intervention. During this phase of the trial, it should be noted that some other factors, like a new illness in a subject, may make the subject ineligible because this new disease might influence the outcome of the clinical trial.

The study is conducted such that one group is treated with the standard treatment available, and the other group is treated with the new drug or treatment under study. If, at some point in the course of the study, the new treatment is thought to be more effective than the standard treatment, the clinical trial is stopped, and all the participants receive the new, more effective treatment. Conversely, if there is any evidence that the new treatment is inferior, toxic, or otherwise harmful, the clinical trial is stopped to protect the patients.

This clinical trial may either be completed or closed when enough people have been treated to satisfy the requirements of the experiment. Still, the final answer may take longer since scientists will continue their observation. Once the drug or treatment has been through the final stage and is found to be safe and effective for human consumption, the FDA or the government authority is likely to approve it to be available for commercial use. On the other hand, though this new drug or treatment may be on the market, researchers still study it for long-term risks or side effects.

Some other points of Phase III clinical trials include the fact that studies at this phase last longer than those of Phase I and II studies. At this phase, placebos, which may be used in some phases of the study, are never used alone if there is a treatment available that works. In most cases, a participant who is assigned to the placebo for part of the clinical trial will, at some point, be offered the standard treatment as well.

Phase IV

During Phase IV of the study, though the FDA has approved the treatment or drug, they are often still watched over a long period. Studies show that though a new treatment or drug might have been tested on thousands of patients, not all the effects may be known. Some of the questions researchers want to answer at this phase are whether there are rare side effects that have not yet been seen. They may also wish to find out if some side effects will show up after a patient has taken this medication for a long time.

Patients can get the treatment or drug used in a Phase IV clinical trial without being part of the study. Normally, the type of care a patient will get in Phase IV of the study will be the care they will get if they are not part of the study. Clinical trials in Phase IV are noted to help scientists learn more about the treatment or drug or provide a service to future patients.

Guinea Pig Myth

There is a common fear within the general population of being used as a guinea pig by researchers. The fear is that their care will be compromised in the name of science. This is not true. As a matter of fact, participants in clinical trials have the best care. There are many specialty doctors on the ground to take care of any eventuality. The patient's well-being is paramount, and these researchers are aware of the privacy concerns. Participants, especially in Phase III, are better placed as far as treatment for their disease is concerned. This is because they will either be receiving the best treatment in the market if they are the control group, or will be receiving experimental therapy with the potential of more effectiveness. The fact that the science community is aware of all these concerns from the general population has made most physicians very sensitive to patients' experiences, the demands of participating in clinical trials, and the need for individualized care for participants. Studies have shown that participating doctors working with experimental therapies give priority to the well-being of the participants over the outcome of the clinical trials.

The Fear of Receiving a Placebo

Studies show that the term placebo is always misleading. Clinical trials are, in most cases, not designed for participants to receive only placebos. Usually, the control group with the placebo will be given standard therapy alone, while the participants in the trial will be given standard treatment, including the clinical trial drug (NCI, 2022). This, therefore, means that all the participants will receive the standard drug while the participants have an addition. If, during the trial, it is realized that the clinical trial drug is more effective, the study will be stopped, and all participants, including the control group, will be treated with the new therapy. Again, most cancer clinical trials do not use placebos unless they are given along with other drugs (NCI, 2022). The only exceptional situation where a placebo alone will be given in a cancer clinical trial is when there is no treatment for that type of cancer.

The Fear of the Side Effects

There is a tendency that all clinical trials will have side effects, and some of them are unknown. But most of these effects are not different from those effects which are mostly usual from the standard treatments, such as hair loss, pain, low blood count, skin burns, especially if it is radiation therapy, nausea, and infection (ACS, 2019). Most of these side effects are temporary. Studies show that there is considerable information known before Phase I of clinical trials. This is because before a drug or therapy is tested on humans, they test them on animals. This makes it easier to know how human beings will tolerate a certain clinical trial. The level of certainty increases from Phases I to III.

The possibility of life-threatening effects from clinical trials can't be ruled out. Some may be permanent, or they may only appear a long time after the treatment is completed. Some of the most serious are those that affect the heart or kidneys. Some of these side effects may only come up after a second cancer or a recurrence. That is why all these side effects must be properly discussed with the patient during the informed consent process, where all questions are answered.

It is, therefore, very important that a participant, together with their doctor and a knowledgeable family member, weighs the risks involved for the participant. The well-being of the patient is paramount. That is why so many questions should be asked, and, if possible, more than one meeting with your healthcare team before a decision is made. In such circumstances, it is equally important to seek a second opinion. In other words, a patient should weigh all the options they have available so they and their family believe they have made the best decision.

Missing out on a Promising Treatment

It is not unusual for doctors to recommend some experimental treatments that are available outside of the clinical trial avenue. This mostly happens if there are promising reports in the early phases of the clinical trials that have not yet been approved, and they offer them as standard treatments (NCI, 2022). Sometimes, patients are tempted to seek this type of treatment because they fear that they might be part of the control group if they participate in clinical trials. This decision might make a patient miss out on a promising treatment they might have had if they had undergone the clinical trial. This unfortunate perception might be because the clinical trial for the treatment is still an ongoing process and has not yet been proven to be better than the current standard of care, and the side effects are not yet conclusive.

On the other hand, despite all the cautions, there may be circumstances where doctors believe the unapproved drug or treatment might be the best for their patients. It is important to note that your doctor does not have an interest in the treatment they are recommending to you. And if they do, then they are not serving the purpose.

The Patient's Advocates

"Should I, as a patient, undergo a clinical trial?" is a question that is difficult to answer immediately. However, most institutions have established a safeguard task force. Although there are no guarantees regarding the outcome of any clinical trials, safeguards are usually in place.

One of the most important parts of this is the Institutional Review Board (IRB). This group is composed of doctors, nurses, scientists, clergy, and a group of knowledgeable laymen and women who are based in the facility where clinical trials are undertaken (NCI, 2022). The responsibility of this group is solely for the protection and welfare of the clinical trial participants in their institution. This group, before the commencement of any clinical trial, examines the potential benefits and risks to the participants. In a nutshell, they examine all aspects of the study. Periodically, while the study is underway, they monitor the data from the clinical trials in their institutions. Cancer studies are also reviewed by the NCI, especially if they are funded by the federal government.

Risks and Benefits

Normally, each clinical trial has some risks and benefits. Studies have shown that clinical trials are more beneficial to the participant for the most part (NCI, 2022). Patients who undergo clinical trials could get a treatment that is not available outside of the clinical trial. This treatment might be better and safer for the patient than any existing current option. By participating in a clinical trial, patients are likely to see their healthcare team more often, who can monitor the progress of their treatment and their disease and be able to check and intervene immediately on the side effects. By participating in a clinical trial, patients take a more active role in their healthcare. In many cases, these trials are funded by the government, which means the financial burden on the patient is often reduced or even eliminated. Participants in clinical trials are helping find a cure for cancer, thus helping other patients who have the same disease and helping to advance cancer research.

Though beneficial to the participants, clinical trials also have some risks. The new treatment tends to have unknown risks that might be worse than those from the standard treatments (NCI, 2022). Participants will have to do a lot of traveling and doctors' visits, which might not be cost-effective, and sometimes, the treatment does not help their disease. Again, participation in clinical trials should be a well-thought-out decision by the participant.

Questions for your Doctor

1. How is this clinical trial beneficial to me, and what will happen to my condition if I don't participate in the trial?

2. I know I will be doing a lot of traveling to the facility where the study is conducted. Who will cover the cost of my transportation?

3. If I happen to fall sick with another illness, will this new illness affect my participation?

4. Can my doctor pick the group I belong to, and will I be able to know which group?

5. If it happens that I have been selected in the control group where I will be given a placebo, can this make my disease worse?

6. How will participating in this study affect my life? Will I be able to continue working and pursue my daily social activities?

7. What are the potential side effects of the clinical trial? Are there long- or short-term effects?

8. Will this study affect my sex life? If so, how?

9. How will I know if the study is working properly for me? Is it possible to receive a different treatment plan if I am not responding well to this study?

10. How much will my personal doctor be involved in this study, and what follow-up care will I have after the study is complete?

11. In a situation where I seem to be harmed during the clinical trial, will I be entitled to care related to the treatment?

12. Who will be professionally responsible for my healthcare while I am in the trial and are my records going to be kept confidential?

13. Who is sponsoring this study, and has it been approved by the federal government agency today and reviewed by the facility board responsible for clinical trials?

CHAPTER 22
Chemotherapy

An aggressive form of chemical drug treatment that kills fast-growing cancer cells in the body is what is often referred to as chemotherapy. At some point in their treatment, most patients receive one or more anticancer agents. These drugs are noted to be the most effective agents that destroy cancer cells because they can reach every part of the body (NCI, 2022). Like some other forms of treatment that are localized in nature, chemotherapy can tackle cancer cells, including those that have metastasized to other parts of the body that are far from the primary site of occurrence. The reason why chemotherapy has this capability is because chemotherapy is injected and spreads through the bloodstream, thus easing its distribution. It is, therefore, considered a systemic treatment because it reaches every part of the body.

Chemotherapy is noted to produce generalized side effects. This is because the whole body is involved in the treatment process. According to studies, chemotherapy is one of the most anxiety-producing forms of treatment because of the expected side effects, which in most cases are not as graphic as the reputation they carry.

Conversely, even if the side effects from the treatment are life-threatening, mechanisms are in place to treat them.

Though the goal of chemotherapy is to destroy fast-dividing cancer cells, some normal cells are also killed. The challenge doctors are facing is how to balance the cancer-destroying benefit of a particular drug or a combination of medications against their toxic effects. Sometimes, it can be such a delicate balance, but with good support and care, the side effects are made tolerable or controlled (ACS, 2019).

How to Prepare for Chemotherapy

Because chemotherapy is a serious treatment, it's important to prepare and plan ahead before starting it. Apart from the fact that a patient must be prepared emotionally, there are a couple of tests a patient must undergo to help determine if they are healthy enough for the treatment. A couple of blood tests are done to determine the health of the liver and the examination of the heart. These tests will also help your oncologist determine the type of chemotherapy drugs to use for your chemotherapy treatment.

It is not unusual for physicians to recommend that their patients visit the dentist before beginning treatment. This is because chemotherapy weakens the body's ability to heal, and any infection in the gums or teeth could potentially spread throughout the body. Since chemotherapy treatment is not a one-time treatment, your doctor may install a port if you are getting the treatment through an intravenous line. This is a device that is implanted in a patient's body, usually on the chest near the shoulder. During each treatment, the IV is inserted into your port. This port allows for easier access to the patient's veins and is less painful.

Now, before the chemotherapy treatment begins, a patient is advised to make work arrangements if they are still employed. Most people can work during their treatment, but they are advised to take on a lighter workload until after the initial couple of sessions to analyze their experiences. Patients are advised to get the help they might need. Getting a friend or relative to help with household activities and taking care of children and pets, if any, will be very helpful as well.

Some of the side effects from chemotherapy treatment, like infertility, can be long-lasting (NCI, 2022). It is important to ask your doctor what side effects you might experience. Patients of childbearing age or those who wish to have children in the future may want to freeze or store eggs, sperm, or fertilized embryos. Patients are advised to join support groups. Talking to someone who has had what you are going through is very important. It will help answer so many questions or concerns and may help you remain optimistic while also helping calm you as a patient of any fears you might have about the treatment.

Ways Chemotherapy Kills Cancer Cells

Patients who undergo chemotherapy may achieve remission, a state in which all signs and symptoms of cancer temporarily disappear or, in some cases, be completely cured. Sometimes, it is used for palliative purposes, which is to relieve pain and symptoms and improve the quality of life for the patient. Chemotherapy may also slow the growth of a tumor, shrink it to make surgical removal easier, or enhance the effectiveness of radiation therapy.

Normally, all cells that are either healthy or abnormal pass through phases in their cycles. These stages include the stage whereby genetic materials or DNA are produced, the meiotic or dividing stage, and the resting stage. A combination of cell cycle-dependent agents that kill cells undergoing cell division and cell cycle-dependent drugs that kill both resting and dividing cells are used. Sometimes, either of the two can be used as well.

Ways of Performing Chemotherapy

Usually, the doctor and the patient will work together, considering all the variables to determine the best course of treatment for their individual cases. Chemotherapy drugs are administered orally, injected into a muscle, under the skin, or intravenously which is into the vein (NCI, 2022). To choose a mode of administration, the doctor will take into consideration the type of cancer, the type of drug to be administered, or the drug combination. For instance, drugs that are in pill form, capsule, or liquid can be taken orally at home, and patients will be making constant visits to the doctor's office for evaluation. Drugs that are not well absorbed by the gastrointestinal tract are injected directly into the bloodstream. Usually, chemotherapy drugs that are given intravenously require a short stay in the facility. It should also be noted that the injectable drugs are done either in a clinic or a doctor's office.

Oral Chemotherapy

Cancer drugs taken orally are more convenient for the patient as well as minimizing cost. As compared to other forms of administration, oral chemotherapy is mostly taken at home and has less toxicity with few side effects (NCI, 2022). One of the main disadvantages of taking chemotherapy drugs orally is the fact that there are many instructions to follow. Some requirements include taking these medications with a lot of water, some on an empty stomach, while others must be taken with food. Patients are usually cautioned to keep records because the consequences might be serious if there is an overdose. That is why most doctors will only prescribe one dose at a time.

Intravenous Chemotherapy

One of the quickest and most popular ways of administering chemotherapy drugs is intravenously (IV). Through this method, chemotherapy drugs are injected into the vein, which will subsequently circulate in the bloodstream and be able to attack cancer cells. This might be accomplished by way of a catheter, pump, or port. Usually, a needle is put in at the beginning of the treatment and removed after the treatment is completed.

By way of a catheter, a thin, soft tube is placed in a large vein, most often in a patient's chest area. The other end of the catheter stays outside in place until a patient finishes their treatment. These catheters are sometimes used for purposes other than the administration of chemotherapy drugs, like drawing blood and administering other medications, such as drugs for pain. Patients are often advised to watch out for infections, especially at the sites.

By way of port or shunt is another method of administering chemotherapy drugs IV. A port, which is either a piece of metal or plastic, is surgically implanted under the patient's skin, usually just below the collar bone or in the upper arm with access to the vein. Drugs are injected into the port with a needle through the skin. The disadvantage of this mode of administration is that there can be a leak of the drug or a shift in the position of the port. Conversely, it has an advantage because it does not require any special care since it is completely under the skin. Patients are always cautioned to watch around the port for signs of infections.

A pump is often attached to the catheter or port to control the flow of the chemotherapy drugs into the patient's veins. The main advantage of using pumps is the fact that they allow patients to receive treatment outside of the hospital setting. Usually, these pumps are either placed externally outside the body or internally under the skin.

Other Forms of Delivery

Sometimes, chemotherapy can be delivered directly into the tumor, depending on the tumor's location. While a patient is undergoing surgery for tumor removal, it is not unusual for the doctor to implant a slowly dissolving disc that releases medication over time. By doing this, larger unusual amounts of drugs are used to destroy cancer cells without affecting surrounding healthy ones. The main advantage of this is that it lowers risks to the patient (NCI, 2022).

Chemotherapy can also be delivered to specific parts of the body through localized treatment. Some common areas of delivery directly include the abdomen, chest, central nervous system, or the bladder through the urethra (NCI, 2022).

Some skin cancers can also be treated with chemotherapy cream. On another note, chemotherapy drugs can also be injected into the muscle or under the skin. This form of administration is rare, though it does allow for slow absorption because some drugs can damage tissues (NCI, 2022).

Intraperitoneal Chemotherapy

This form of chemotherapy delivery is mostly used when delivering drugs into the abdominal cavity or peritoneum. Usually, a catheter is placed in the abdominal cavity on a special device worn on the chest or abdomen. A chamber is filled with drugs that flow through the catheter into the abdominal cavity. Ovarian cancer is best treated with this mode (NCI, 2022).

Intravesical Chemotherapy

This mode of delivery is intended to deliver chemotherapy directly into the bladder to treat bladder cancer. Usually, a catheter is inserted into the bladder for one to three hours while drugs flow through into the bladder. This form of chemotherapy is mostly done by a urologist on an outpatient basis. To make sure the drug reaches all parts of the bladder, the patient shifts position every 15 minutes.

Intraventricular and Intrathecal Chemotherapy

This is a situation whereby chemotherapy drugs are placed directly into the spinal fluid. It is mostly used to treat metastatic cancers of the brain and spinal cord. Usually, the drug is either injected directly into the spinal cord, known as intrathecal chemotherapy, or placed in a rubber bulb or Ommaya reservoir that allows the drug to flow directly into the brain, a process known as intraventricular chemotherapy. Usually, a surgeon implants the bulb under the patient's scalp and threads a small catheter into the ventricle of the brain. Chemotherapy drugs can then be injected into the reservoir. This helps to avoid the repeated injections necessary to deliver the drug to the spinal fluid that flows over the brain continuously.

Side Effects

Chemotherapy drugs do not know the difference between healthy and cancer cells. This, therefore, means that the treatment affects healthy cells as well, especially those that are rapidly dividing. Studies show that healthy cells in the mouth, stomach, intestine, and hair follicles are susceptible to temporary damage from chemotherapy treatment. It is noted that chemotherapy drugs can cause some serious toxic effects on the bone marrow, heart, and kidney (NCI, 2022). It is, therefore, important that a patient undergoing chemotherapy treatment should be monitored closely and carefully with treatment plan changes if the need arises. Patients who experience some of these toxic effects are susceptible to lower resistance to infection or damage to vital organs.

The fact that people have inherent differences and variations in health, their experiences with chemotherapy treatment differ as well with different side effects. In addition, each chemotherapy drug or a combination of drugs will have a different side effect. Studies show that most chemotherapy drugs have more than one side effect, with an increase in intensity and variations as treatment progresses. The good thing about it is that most of the side effects are temporary and there are ways of resolving them.

Leakages

The leakage of chemotherapy drugs from a vein into nearby healthy tissue is one of the risks of this type of treatment. This does not happen most of the time, but it's something to watch out for. Some of the signs include stinging, burning, or swelling around the area where the drug was injected. It is noted that within a couple of days, the area becomes inflamed and painful. Subsequently, ulceration and other damages might affect the functions of nerves and tendons around the area. Again, leakages are not usual but should be reported immediately to your healthcare team and they will be treated or changes made accordingly.

Nausea and Vomiting

Nausea and vomiting are noted to be two of the most common side effects of chemotherapy. Unfortunately, the exact causes of chemotherapy-induced vomiting and nausea are not fully understood. From all indications, certain areas of the brain are being triggered during treatment. When these parts of the brain are triggered, they activate a reflex, causing the sensation of nausea and vomiting. Chemotherapy treatments are noted to cause vomiting and nausea when given in large quantities. On the other hand, it is not unusual to be mildly nauseated or vomiting with even small quantities of drug intake (Murphy, G.P., Morris, L.B., & Lange, D., 1997).

Usually, nausea and vomiting start a few hours after treatment and last for a few hours as well. But sometimes, there is anticipatory nausea and vomiting, which happens before treatment. This can occur as a learned response that develops because of previous chemotherapy treatments that led to nausea and vomiting. Less often, severe nausea and vomiting can last for up to two days, which might lead to dehydration and loss of appetite. There are many combinations of drugs given to people undergoing treatment to prevent and control nausea and vomiting. Nausea and vomiting must be overcome so that the body gets the energy it needs to recover from the effects of the drugs.

Research equally shows that about half of the people receiving chemotherapy feel queasy even before the treatment begins and sometimes vomit before receiving any drugs (NCI, 2022). Again, this anticipation is not unusual, and it is noted to be triggered by the smell of the treatment room where a patient might have had a previous treatment, the hospital or clinic, or even the sight of the hospital. The best way to handle this nausea is through a simple relaxation technique, such as imagining a pleasant scene like a beach, a nice party you attended, a good encounter with a loved one, or what you like. Focusing on previous good experiences is a good distraction, which is very helpful.

Hair Loss

Hair loss may be one of the most devastating side effects of chemotherapy. This is because it seems like a great violation of a healthy appearance. Also, not all chemotherapy drugs cause hair loss. People have different intensities of hair loss. Some might be mild, while some might be very severe to the extent of losing every hair on their body, including the head, armpits, legs, eyebrows, eyelashes, and even pubic hairs.

Usually, hair loss does not happen immediately. It might take a few weeks during or after treatment. It might start falling out from the roots and eventually into clumps. As harsh as it may sound, there are ways of coping with this.

Patients are always advised to contact a hair stylist before beginning their chemotherapy treatment. Most of the time, their hair will be cut short, and this helps to prepare their minds regarding what to expect during and after their treatment. While on treatment, patients are advised to handle their hair gently, comb carefully without pulling, and not use wash chemicals such as hair dyes or permanent waving products.

For those who plan to wear a wig, it is advisable to get one before beginning treatment. By buying ahead of time, they will be able to match their natural hair color and desired style. It is not unusual for patients to cover their hair with a hat, scarf, or wig once their hair starts coming out. In most cases, it is very difficult for people to see them losing their hair. It can be traumatizing, especially if the hair falls out in clumps. Though it might take a long time to get back your hair, in most cases patients will always have it back. The other good news is that the hair might look better and thicker.

Mucositis

Mucositis happens to be one of those serious side effects of chemotherapy treatment that causes bleeding, sores, and pain in the mouth and throat of the patient. In most cases, the mouth is dry and susceptible to infection. Mucositis is noted to sometimes make everyday tasks such as eating and drinking difficult and, in some cases, impossible. Precautionary measures are recommended to minimize this side effect. An increase in the number of times patients brush their teeth, regular dental exams, keeping your mouth moisturized, and not smoking are some helpful tips. Patients are also advised to eat their foods cold or at room temperature and avoid acidic, spicy, or salty foods (ACS, 2019). In extreme situations where a patient can't eat, they may be fed by way of a feeding tube. Finally, mucositis is noted to subside or get better a few weeks after chemotherapy treatment. On the other hand, if it gets worse, your healthcare team will always prescribe relieving medications.

Diarrhea

Diarrhea is another side effect that can occur from chemotherapy treatment. It occurs when the chemotherapy drugs affect the lining of the intestine. When this occurs, your doctor will recommend medications to resolve the problem. Recently, over-the-counter medications and prescriptions have become available. Patients are advised to always consult with their healthcare team for any eventualities.

Fatigue

Fatigue is a common side effect of chemotherapy treatment, which can be mild or severe. Sometimes, a patient may feel completely wiped out. This happens because the body is fighting the effects of the chemotherapy drugs and trying to recover from the dead, lost cells, thereby giving up a lot of energy. It is also noted that fatigue comes about because of anemia or loss of red blood cells, which are known to carry oxygen to the body tissues.

From experience, fatigue tends to be more severe at the beginning of the treatment and declines in intensity toward the end. However, it gets progressively worse as the number of cycles increases (NCI, 2022). The good news is that it gradually disappears at the end of the treatment. Patients are always advised to listen to their bodies to fight fatigue. Patients should not push themselves to do activities that might require a lot of energy. That is why help from family and friends is recommended. Another recommendation is that the energy-required activities should be reserved for when the patient is most energetic and should have scheduled intervals between treatments. When planning for your treatment sessions, factor in fatigue.

Sex and Fertility

Chemotherapy affects a patient's sex and fertility both directly and indirectly. Other side effects from chemotherapy treatment, like nausea and fatigue, are equally noted to lower a patient's libido as well. Also, since patients lose their hair when they are undergoing chemotherapy treatment, they believe they are less attractive to their partners, thus a decrease in their desire. It is also noted that the stomach upset and weakness from the chemotherapy treatment reduce both the emotional and the physical desire for sexual activity. Most people find their sexual desire returns after the side effects of the treatment go away. On the other hand, people find it very frustrating because, by the time they start developing sexual desire, they are ready for another cycle of treatment. Again, the good news is that people return to sexual normality after completing their treatment.

As far as the sexes are concerned, studies show that in men, some situations of permanent effects on erections exist after chemotherapy treatment (NCI, 2022). This is because some chemotherapy drugs do affect nerves that control erection. On the other hand, most men exhibit erections throughout their treatment. There are also situations whereby men exhibit dry orgasms. This is when chemotherapy damages the nerves controlling the emission of semen. In this situation, the male may feel pleasure, but no semen comes out during ejaculation. Patients are advised to have a discussion with their healthcare team before treatment because it might be traumatizing to a lot of people, especially those who are still very sexually active.

For women, the female reproductive organs, especially the ovaries, are very sensitive to chemotherapy. Sometimes, menstrual periods are interrupted during chemotherapy treatment. At this point, it is not unusual to either have short or prolonged menstrual flows. Menopause-like symptoms such as vaginal dryness, hot flashes, and night sweats are not unusual during treatment. The long-term effects of the female menstrual cycle or proper functioning of the organs after treatment differ from person to person. Some women, especially those who are near menopause, may go into permanent menopause. While some women of childbearing age might regain their fertility, there is a likelihood that they might not be fertile again or be able to bear children. Women of childbearing age or who want to have children in the future are always advised to freeze their eggs before starting their chemotherapy treatment. Having a thorough discussion with your healthcare team and asking as many questions as you can is very helpful.

Pregnancy

The fact that chemotherapy causes infertility in both men and women does not mean that a woman can't get pregnant when they are undergoing chemotherapy treatment. The issue about it is that it is risky to both the fetus and the woman. More than that, the physical changes because of the pregnancy compound the side effects of the treatment. The chances of birth defects in the baby are high, though not in all cases.

For women who were already pregnant before their cancer diagnosis, it is advisable to postpone their chemotherapy treatment till after delivery. It is not unusual to delay the treatment until after the twelfth week of pregnancy when the fetus might be at less risk of the chemotherapy drugs (NCI, 2022). All of these concerns have to be discussed with your doctor before the start of the treatment.

Effects on Emotions

Nobody wants to be sick, and based on experiences and research, the strain of being sick, coupled with the side effects and the devastation that chemotherapy drugs might bring on one's body, may take a toll on a patient's well-being. Chemotherapy is noted to make patients feel angry, depressed, afraid, and anxious. It can be emotionally draining, especially since you have to change your routine. All one's appointments revolve around their chemotherapy treatment timetable, sometimes including work schedules. It is not unusual for patients to forgo some of their enjoyable activities like sports, parties, etc., because of fatigue and even lack of taste for food. It is also known that some people, while on chemotherapy treatment, may face confusion, memory loss, unconsciousness, and even agitation (NCI, 2022).

These emotional swings and physiological changes, which are anticipated side effects, can be very scary to the patient who is about to start their chemotherapy treatment. That is why patients are advised to talk about their fears to family, friends, and some support groups or people who have been in the situation they are about to get into. The good news is that the cognitive and emotional effects will subside after the chemotherapy treatment.

Weakened Immune System

Patients undergoing chemotherapy treatment have their immune system compromised. This is because chemotherapy drugs significantly lower white blood cell count. White blood cells are very vital to the immune system, and when a low white blood cell count occurs, it makes it harder for the immune system to fight off bacteria, viruses, and some other pathogens. The fact that the immune system is compromised increases the risk of infection.

Most often, people whose immune system is compromised exhibit the following symptoms, which include fever, chills, difficulty breathing, rectal and abdominal pain, and cough (ACS, 2019). Patients undergoing chemotherapy treatment are advised to take steps to avoid getting sick. Regular hand washing, avoiding crowded places, and staying away from people who may make them sick will help decrease the rate of infection. Good food preparation is also recommended. This helps to reduce food poisoning. While your doctor might recommend antibiotics to help reduce this, if it persists, the treatment can be delayed temporarily to allow the body to make the most needed white blood cells.

Nail Changes

Most patients who undergo chemotherapy treatment experience changes in their nails. These mostly permanent changes can create discoloration, dryness, and blemishes. It is not unusual for nails to look bruised, and sometimes, they may turn black, brown, or blue or become abnormally thin or brittle. In some situations, the nail might fall off completely.

There is usually a high probability of infection when nail changes do occur. That is why it is very important to have your nails trimmed and cleaned during and after your chemotherapy treatment. People who are experiencing this situation are equally encouraged to decrease the risk of infection by wearing gloves, especially when they are cleaning or doing any form of manual labor. Having your nails painted will also be helpful to strengthen your nails. Patients are also advised to avoid picking and biting their nails.

Effects on Bone Marrow

Bone marrow is an integral part of human health which produces three types of blood cells that are vulnerable to chemotherapy because they are constantly dividing. These include red blood cells, which carry oxygen throughout the body; white blood cells, which fight infection; and platelets, which help blood clot or stop bleeding. All these blood cells should be monitored closely because a drop of any of them could have a very serious effect.

Usually, the treatment team performs a blood test for blood count at the beginning of each cycle and later between a week and 10 days (NCI, 2022). During this period, white blood cells and platelets are noted to be at the lowest level, leaving the body vulnerable to infection.

Side Effects on Muscle and Nerve

Sometimes, chemotherapy treatment affects the nervous system, a condition known as peripheral neuropathy (NCI, 2022). When this happens, a patient will have the following symptoms: burning, weakness, tingling, numbness of hands or feet, or both. In a situation when the nerves are affected, a patient may experience jaw pain, loss of balance, hearing loss, stomach pain, constipation, and difficulty walking. When muscles are affected, a patient may feel weak, sore, or tired. Like every other side effect or concern, patients are advised to inform their healthcare team immediately.

Other Side Effects

Sometimes, patients who are on chemotherapy treatment can have some mental changes, which are either short or long-term (ACS, 2019). It is not unusual for these patients to have a hard time remembering certain words or memories, learning new skills, or concentrating on tasks. Some of these patients might not remember some names or words. To help alleviate this, patients are advised to undergo cognitive rehabilitation activities to help improve brain function, as well as meditation and exercise.

It is also not unusual for patients to gain weight following their chemotherapy treatment. This happens mostly in women who have had chemotherapy for breast cancer. While watching your weight, patients are advised not to overstrain themselves, especially by dieting.

Footnotes

Studies show that most of the side effects from chemotherapy treatment subside. On the other hand, some side effects, like infertility, menstrual changes, organ damage, and low white blood cell count, may last longer (NCI, 2022). Based on the fact that a patient might have had bad experiences when they were undergoing their chemotherapy treatment, they develop a lot of anxiety and even fear of the return of the disease. Patients are encouraged to join support groups with other people who have had similar experiences. Friends and family are usually advised to be very supportive and not to expect a lot from some of the relations because things might not be the same for them.

Questions for your Doctor

1. What are the side effects of chemotherapy treatment?

2. Will I be able to have children after my chemotherapy treatment?

3. If my cancer returns or I have another cancer, will I be able to have chemotherapy for this second cancer?

4. For the organs that might be damaged because of chemotherapy treatment, is there a possibility they may regain their functionality, or will this be permanent damage?

5. What might be the consequences if I refuse chemotherapy treatment?

6. Will I be able to regain my full energy potential after the treatment?

7. What food or diet do you recommend for me after my chemotherapy treatment?

8. Since chemotherapy drugs might be toxic, will this affect people around me?

9. Will I be able to function normally, including work and social activities, during my chemotherapy treatment?

10. Will I be able to drive during my treatment?

11. How long will the side effects last, especially those that are long-term?

CHAPTER 23
Radiation Therapy

Radiation therapy happens to be one of the most common methods of cancer treatment. This form of treatment uses high doses of radiation to kill cancer cells and shrink tumors. Radiation therapy is also known as radiotherapy, irradiation, and X-ray therapy. It is used in a variety of ways, alone or combined with other therapies such as chemotherapy or surgery. This mode of treatment comes in different forms, which include X-rays or photons, gamma rays, electron beams, and protons, all aimed at solving the same problem with different intensities based on the location, stage, size of the cancer, size of the patient and what the doctor wishes to accomplish.

Radiation works by making small breaks in the DNA inside cells. These breaks keep cancer cells from growing and dividing, thus causing the cells to die. Radiation therapy also affects normal cells, but most of the normal cells recover and return to their original working functions (ACS, 2019). Vulnerable areas of the body are shielded during the treatment so they are not exposed unnecessarily. Most patients usually have the concern of unnecessary exposure, which is a vital concern. Still, it should be noted that the concern is usually taken into consideration during the treatment planning and delivery process. Radiation therapy alone can cure cancer, depending on the stage. Conversely, it is also used for palliative purposes, to relieve pain and symptoms, or to prevent further complications. Palliative radiation therapy, for example, can shrink a tumor that is causing pressure and pain because it is impinging on nerves and nearby organs.

Radiation for Cancer Treatment

Radiation is noted to be a primary treatment for certain cancers that are vulnerable to this type of treatment. Examples of such cancers include most forms of head and neck cancers, Hodgkin's disease, and non-Hodgkin lymphomas, lungs, breast, cervix, bladder, thyroid, prostate, testes, and brain (ACS, 2019). It is also used to damage cells that have spread to other parts of the body. Sometimes, patients who are about to have bone marrow transplant have their whole body irradiated before the transplant.

Radiation Therapy as Primary Treatment

Radiation therapy, unlike other forms of treatment like chemotherapy, which requires exposing the entire body to cancer-fighting drugs, affects only the tumor and the surrounding area, usually a couple of inches. It is noted that radiation and surgery have similar cure rates for certain types of cancers. Radiation therapy is sometimes preferred to surgery if a patient has a preexisting condition that makes surgery challenging or if surgery may require the removal of a limb or an organ. In such circumstances, radiation therapy is often chosen to preserve normal organs and to keep the body fully functional. A prime example of a situation where radiation is preferred over other forms of treatment is to preserve a patient's voice in the treatment of cancer of the larynx (ACS, 2019).

Radiation Therapy as a Combined Treatment

To enhance the curing of cancer, radiation therapy is frequently combined with other forms of treatment, mostly surgery and chemotherapy. Sometimes, radiation may be administered before the removal of a tumor to kill the outermost cancer cells, which could dislodge and spread during the operation. In some cases, radiation may be used to shrink the tumor so that it can be surgically removed more easily or to make the operation less radical, thereby preserving the nearby tissues.

Radiation therapy is sometimes recommended after surgery, which is aimed at killing cancer cells that were not easily removed or where cancer cells may remain. The treatment of the breast with radiation therapy after surgery or lumpectomy is a good example. The duration between surgery and when to start the radiation treatment depends on how fast a patient is recuperating. It could be a couple of days or weeks after surgery.

The combination of chemotherapy and radiation therapy can be a helpful addition. In most cases, these two modes of treatment are administered to patients after surgery. The rationale for this is to get rid of any remaining cancer cells in the body. Chemotherapy chemicals may work by rendering cancer cells more radiosensitive, by independently killing cells, or by enhancing the effects of radiation therapy, studies show (NCI, 2022).

Types of Radiation Therapy

There are mainly two types of radiation therapy: external beam radiation, which directs radiation from outside sources into the body, and internal therapy, also known as brachytherapy, in which a radioactive source is placed inside the body, near the growth area.

The type of radiation therapy that a patient may have depends on a couple of factors, including the type of cancer, size of the tumor, location, general health and medical history of the patient, age, and whether the patient has other types of cancer treatment.

External Beam Radiation Therapy

External beam radiation therapy comes from radiation equipment that emits radiation aimed at radiating a patient's cancer. A huge machine that emits this radiation is placed a couple of feet from the patient, though sometimes the distance to the patient may be shorter. It rotates around the patient, but it will not touch them. External beam radiation therapy happens to be a local treatment, which means that it treats a specific part of the body. This includes head and neck, prostate, breast, lung, etc.

The above-mentioned parts of the body, including many others, are treated using high-energy or megavoltage radiation. This is because high energy is strong enough to penetrate most internal organs and structures and to shrink deep tumors. It is important to note that high-energy radiation does not attain its full strength until it reaches some planned depth in the body. This, therefore, means that the skin and tissues close to the skin receive mild radiation, which usually causes only minor and temporary side effects. Also, the radiation beam is often directed from more than one angle so that the radiation is focused on the tumor, thus sparing all but a small margin of surrounding normal tissues. The frequency of treatment is mostly Monday through Friday, though sometimes every other day in case of hyperfractionation.

Low-energy or orthovoltage radiation, on the other hand, does not penetrate very deeply into the body and is used mainly to treat surface cancers such as skin cancer. The prescription of external beam radiation may last for about five to six weeks of continuous treatment, except on weekends. This schedule prevents the skin and normal tissues from receiving too much radiation at a time and equally enables the patient to recuperate. It is also not unusual to administer radiation two or three times a week, especially on slow-growing cancers like that of the skin, for three to five weeks, especially if the intent is to alleviate symptoms (ACS, 2019). In some situations, split-course therapy is prescribed, which allows the body time to recover from minor side effects. The question that often arises from patients is whether one or two days of non-continuous radiation treatment will affect the outcome of the treatment. In most cases, it isn't because a couple of missed days are added at the end of the course, but it is always necessary to talk to your doctor or healthcare team about such concerns.

Another form of external beam radiation administered during surgery in the operating room is known as intraoperative radiation therapy. This makes it possible to deliver a large dose of radiation to tumors without harming healthy tissues in the path of the beam. The aim of using this type of radiation treatment is a preventive measure to destroy stray cancer cells that may proliferate even though the initial tumor has been removed.

Stereotactic radiation therapy is among other types of external beam radiation therapy. Currently, this type of external beam radiation therapy is used to treat mostly cancers of the brain and prostate. However, as technology evolves, it will be able to treat other sites. A robotic arm targets the tumor from a couple of directions while minimizing the exposure of the surrounding tissues.

Proton radiation therapy happens to be a new technology in the treatment of cancer. Unlike traditional radiation that uses photons that penetrate the body, proton therapy targets solid tumors with pinpoint accuracy. It delivers a maximum radiation dose that stops at the tumor site while sparing healthy surrounding tissues, unlike other forms of external beam therapies. There are usually a few side effects, including secondary cancers caused by radiation. Though photons and protons might be similar in that they both destroy cancer cells, protons have the advantage of depositing little radiation and stopping at the tumor site. Another advantage of proton therapy is the fact that long-term side effects are minimized comparatively (NCI, 2022).

Internal Radiation Therapy

Sometimes, radioactive material is placed inside the body near a tumor to deliver radiation to the tumor. This is referred to as internal radiation therapy. This radioactive material is sometimes inserted into the body, injected, or swallowed into a special solution. Examples of the most common radiation sources are iridium, cesium, iodine, phosphorus, and gold. These are all sources that give up low-energy radiation, which makes it easier to spare the surrounding healthier tissues. Radiation delivered internally is advantageous because more radiation can be delivered to the target within a short time than with the external beam. Another advantage of this form of radiation is the fact that the source of the radiation is so close to the cancer cells, which minimizes unnecessary radiation to healthy tissues.

Internal radiation is, in most cases, often used as an adjunct to external beam radiation. It sometimes acts as a boost. Another name for internal radiation therapy is brachytherapy. Other names include systemic therapy, which means that the treatment travels in the blood to tissues throughout a patient's body and kills cancer cells. Like other forms of liquid medications, a patient receives systemic radiation therapy by swallowing, through a vein via an IV line, or through an injection. It is noted that with systemic radiation, a patient's body fluids, such as urine, sweat, and saliva, will give off radiation for a while (NCI, 2022). That is why patients undergoing this type of treatment are either contained in a room or shielded to prevent unnecessary exposure to the public.

Goals of Radiation Therapy

Though radiation therapy is often prescribed for cancer treatment, most types of radiation therapy don't reach all parts of the body. This implies that it will not be helpful in treating cancer that has spread to many parts of the body. But though it might have small limitations, it can be used to treat many types of cancer either alone or in combination with other forms of treatment. The prescription for radiation treatment might be different from one form of cancer to another and from patient to patient because they are all different. The choice of treatment will depend on what the doctor wants to accomplish.

To cure or shrink cancer

Certain types of cancers are noted to be very sensitive to radiation. In such circumstances, radiation may be used to shrink or cure. In some other cases, chemotherapy or other cancer drugs may be given first. For some cancers, radiation therapy is used before surgery to shrink the tumor or after surgery to help keep the cancer from returning.

It is noted that for cancers that can be cured either by surgery or radiation therapy, radiation is preferred. This is because there is less damage to the area, and the part of the body involved is more likely to perform its original functions normally (NCI, 2022).

Studies show that for some types of cancer, radiation therapy and chemotherapy might be used together. Certain drugs are known to help radiation work better by making cancer cells more sensitive to radiation therapy. It is noted that when anti-cancer drugs and radiation are given together for some types of cancers, they complement each other and even work better than if they were given individually. The downside of this combination is the fact that the side effects are worse (ACS, 2019).

To stop recurrence
Cancer tends to spread to other parts of the body away from where it started. In some cases, the area where the cancer most often spreads might be treated with radiation to kill any cancer cells before they grow into tumors. It is not unusual to give radiation to an adjacent part of the body at the same time radiation is given in an affected area. This is because there is a likelihood of cancer spreading to this close area.

To treat symptoms
It is not unusual for cancer to spread to other parts of the body, which might be due to poor treatment when it was initially diagnosed or it had already spread before it was discovered. Radiation therapy can be used to treat these tumors to make them smaller. Sometimes, radiation therapy is given for palliative purposes, especially if the cancer is already advanced or has spread to other parts of the body.

The goal at this point is to alleviate problems like pain, trouble breathing or swallowing, or bowel obstruction because of advanced disease (NCI, 2022).

To treat recurrence

When cancer returns, radiation therapy might be used to treat the cancer or the symptoms caused by the cancer. Radiation may be considered again in the same area if the tissue has not already received its maximum allowable dose during previous treatment. However, if the maximum dose has already been reached, repeating radiation in that area may not be a safe or effective option. Still, in some cases, retreatment might be recommended if the potential benefits outweigh the risks of doing nothing.

Radiation Therapy as a Cause for Another Cancer

Studies show that there is a probability of developing another cancer after receiving radiation therapy aimed at treating your disease (ACS, 2019). This is the one possible side effect doctors or your healthcare team have to take into consideration before prescribing radiation therapy to treat your cancer. Evidence suggests low doses of radiation increase cancer incidence (NCI, 2022). This side effect is very crucial to the extent that doctors should weigh the risks and benefits associated with each mode of treatment at their disposal. For the most part, the risk of developing a second cancer after receiving radiation therapy is very small, and it is more beneficial to the patient. Still, it can't be ruled out completely. Leukemia is noted to be one of those cancers that are caused by radiation, which typically shows up 10 or more years after the initial radiation therapy treatment. Other forms of cancers that are caused by radiation therapy are thyroid and breast cancers, usually fifteen years after the first radiation treatment (NCI, 2022). Note that the risk is different depending on the area of treatment.

Based on the stage of the cancer and the part of the body involved, if your doctor recommends radiation therapy for your condition, know the benefits outweigh the risks. Not all radiation treatments will cause cancer, but the risk might be dependent on a couple of factors. The younger a person is when they receive radiation treatment, the greater the risk of developing another cancer sometime later in their life. It is also noted from studies that the type of disease such as Hodgkin's has a higher probability of the patient developing cancer after radiation treatment (ACS, 2019). Though it might sound risky, the benefit of treating your cancer with radiation therapy outweighs the opposite effect of not treating the disease using this mode of treatment for fear of developing another cancer in the future where the probability is low.

Diet While on Radiation Therapy

Radiation therapy is noted to cause a change in a patient's appetite due to side effects, which include nausea, mouth sores, and throat problems (NCI, 2022). It is important to eat enough calories and protein to maintain your weight and energy during treatment since your body uses a lot of energy to heal during your radiation therapy treatment. For people who are having trouble eating and maintaining their weight, it is advisable to talk to your doctor or healthcare team about your condition. Your doctor or provider might recommend that you see a dietician.

Again, it is common for a patient receiving radiation therapy not to feel like eating, but it is important to overcome this temporary loss of appetite. Remember, your body is losing energy due to the radiation treatment and now needs more calories and nutrients. According to studies, the trick is to eat as much as you can when you are very hungry. In a nutshell, take advantage of every situation you might have at your disposal as much as possible.

Most people have a regular eating habit, such as eating three times a day at certain periods of the day. But now that they are in this situation, they should learn to eat even when they are not hungry, even if it is not a regular mealtime and even if it means eating several smaller meals rather than three big meals each day. It is important to have snacks such as frozen yogurt, fruits, fruit juice, and high-calorie snacks and nutritional supplements, especially if a patient is losing weight (ACS, 2019). Other ways by which a patient can increase their appetite is by making their meals pleasurable, such as eating with friends, playing good music while eating, and making sure they eat what they desire. As always, if a patient is having trouble eating or maintaining their weight, it is advisable to talk to their doctor or healthcare team for recommendations.

Skin Care

Skin reaction happens to be one of the main side effects of radiation therapy treatment. (See side effects). How to overcome this side effect is always of great concern to most patients, especially women. Due to technical advancement, the amount of radiation absorbed by the skin has greatly reduced, though the area irradiated will always have a local reaction. Here are some recommendations, but it is always advisable to talk to your healthcare team with any concerns.

When taking a shower, patients are advised to wash the skin in the treatment area with warm water. Instead of rubbing the area as they would normally do when showering, they should pat it dry with warm water while making sure not to take off the skin markings made by the radiation team. For those who wish to use soap while showering, mild and unscented soaps are recommended (ACS, 2019).

Patients are advised not to use lotions, perfumes, creams, powder deodorant, makeup, or alcohol-containing skin products on the affected area, except as prescribed by the doctor (ACS, 2019). This is because some of these products might have a reactive effect on the patient's skin. Some of these effects include rashes, dry and wet decimation, and wounds. In situations of this nature, the doctor will prescribe remedies, or sometimes patients take breaks from the radiation treatment.

Patients are encouraged to wear protective clothing in cold weather and to avoid sunlight on the treatment areas especially when they are still receiving treatment. If possible, patients should apply sunscreens or blocks if they cannot cover the affected area during and after treatment because the area will remain sensitive during this period.

Do not use heating pads, hot water bottles, cold packs, or heating lamps on the affected area (ACS, 2019). Equally, wear loose-fitting clothing over the area exposed to radiation. Though patients are always advised to inform their doctor, the nurse, or the therapist of any side effects, the good thing is that since mostly the same therapists are administering the treatment, in case of any unusual effect, they will notice and report to the doctor.

Side Effects from Radiation Therapy Treatment

Most people receiving radiation therapy will have some side effects from the treatment. Although significant efforts are being made to prevent the radiation from impacting normal tissues, some contact is unavoidable, which will eventually lead to some side effects. It is also important to note that not every case is the same, so people react differently to the treatment. Normally, the side effects someone might have depend on the type and location of the cancer, the dose of radiation given, and the patient's general health. Some of these side effects are general, while others are specific to the area being treated. Some people have fewer or no side effects, while others are unlucky. Though most of these side effects are temporary, there are some long-term effects, and there are ways to handle them as well.

How Long Do the Side Effects Last

Among other factors, the type of side effects a patient may experience can depend on the prescribed dose and the treatment schedule. Most side effects go away within a couple of months after the end of the radiation treatment, but some are long-term.

Some side effects might limit a patient's ability to do certain things, though that may depend on how a patient feels. Some people can do most of their activities, like leisure and going to work, while they are undergoing their radiation therapy treatment. Some patients, on the other hand, prefer to rest after their daily treatment, which can be energy-draining. Patients are always advised to inform their healthcare team about any side effects. For any eventualities regarding side effects, the doctor will change the prescription, change the schedule, or stop the treatment. Stopping the treatment at a certain point might not make any difference regarding your care. But this decision must be made by your doctor with your involvement.

Fatigue

Fatigue or tiredness is one of the most common side effects of radiation therapy treatment experienced by more than 90% of the patients on treatment (ACS, 2019). The level of fatigue is sometimes based on the size of the area and the location being treated. Patients having treatment in their abdominal area experience more fatigue than the rest of the population. The level of fatigue increases proportionate to the increase in the number of times a patient receives treatment. Studies show that tiredness is more intense between the fourth and the fifth weeks of treatment (NCI, 2022). The cause of fatigue could be the fact that both healthy and cancer cells are being destroyed during treatment and the stress from the daily trips to the treatment center. It could also be that the healing process drains a lot of energy.

Studies show that fatigue due to radiation therapy treatment is different from fatigue from everyday life. It also shows that it might not get better with rest, and that is why managing it is an important part of the care. Sometimes, it can last a long time and can get in the way of individual routine activities, but it subsides a couple of weeks after the end of the treatment. Now, it is only you who knows the level of your fatigue, so you must notify your healthcare team about how you feel so they will be able to help you with your situation. Most patients on radiation therapy treatment will take a break from work because it is very draining to handle both.

Skin Problems

Usually, the skin in the radiated area undergoes some changes that might look red, dry, and itchy. It can equally be swollen, irritated, or tanned. It is not unusual for your skin to start peeling off (radiation dermatitis). Another form of skin reaction that may occur is moist desquamation, a situation in which the skin folds, especially under the breast for breast treatment or by the hip joint for patients who are receiving treatment in their pelvic area. (See skin care above on how to manage this side effect.)

Hair Loss

Patients undergoing radiation therapy treatment will, at some point, lose their hair in the area of treatment. This is most pronounced among patients who are having treatment around their head and neck area. It is not unusual for hair to start falling off the head, eyebrows, and lashes. Though not noticed by the public, patients lose their hair in the pubic area, too, if that part of the body is being treated with radiation. What will not happen is hair loss in an area that is not being treated with radiation, except if a patient is having a combined treatment with another therapy such as chemotherapy. From experience, most patients' hair grows back, although it might be thinner or have a different texture from the way it was before, which might be difficult for some people to bear.

Now, for those who have hair loss on their head, it is advisable to cover their head since their scalp may be tender to prevent exposure to the sun. For those who prefer to wear artificial hair or wigs, make sure the lining does not affect or irritate your scalp. Always talk to your healthcare team about any concerns. Beauty shops and spas may be helpful in finding something artificial that might help preserve your looks. Again, most hair loss is temporary and will always grow back (ACS, 2019).

Mouth Dryness and Sore Throat

It is not unusual for some symptoms to come about as a response to the organ or structure being treated. People respond differently to the radiation. Consequently, patients will have different experiences.

Though these experiences are mostly temporary, in some cases, they might last for years. When a patient is radiated in the head and neck area, it is not unusual for the mucous membrane of the mouth to become red, experience extreme dryness of the mouth and lips, and have difficulty swallowing. Some people lose their sense of taste, especially if the tongue is in the area of treatment. The salivary gland might be affected, too; thus, they will not be able to produce the required amount of saliva. I have had a couple of patients whose voices have been affected for a couple of years but with a gradual recovery.

Among some of the remedies recommended to solve this problem, patients are advised to drink a lot of water and suck hard candy, which might help provide some relief (ACS, 2019). On the other hand, patients are equally advised not to use alcohol-containing mouthwash because it can intensify the radiation reaction. Patients are also advised not to smoke or drink alcohol while on treatment. In most cases, during consultation, the doctor will recommend that patients see the dentist before beginning radiation treatment. Patients are advised to rinse their mouth with warm soda water and salt every other hour, moisten food with gravies to eat, and sip cool drinks often throughout the day (ACS, 2019).

Low Blood Count

Though rare, radiation therapy can cause changes in a patient's blood count level. Normally, these blood cells help a patient's body fight infection while helping to prevent bleeding. Some symptoms of low blood count include weakness. Sometimes, treatment is interrupted if a patient experiences a low blood count, at least temporarily, to allow the count to get back to normal.

Nausea and Vomiting

Nausea and vomiting are common side effects of radiation therapy treatment. This affects mostly patients who are having radiation treatment around the abdominal and pelvic area. Sometimes, doctors recommend that anti-nausea medication be taken before and after every treatment session. Other effects associated with radiation around the abdominal area are diarrhea, cramping, gassiness, and bloating (ACS, 2019). Though over-the-counter medications can be okay for your diarrhea, it is recommended that you talk to your healthcare team about any abnormality.

Pregnancy and Fertility

Female: Infertility is noted to be one of the long-term side effects, especially if a person is receiving radiation treatment around the abdominal and pelvic area. It is not unusual for women to experience difficulties becoming pregnant, stop menstruating, and even experience symptoms of menopause. Infertility may be permanent in some cases, though it might be possible to prevent sterility by shielding the ovaries during treatment, but I wouldn't take a chance. Women of childbearing age are advised not to conceive during their radiation treatment because it might be harmful to the developing fetus. For those who wish to have children later in life, you must discuss with your doctor how it might affect the possibility of having children in the future.

Men: Men whose testicles are radiated usually have a reduction in the sperm count, the ability to fertilize an egg will diminish, and sometimes it might lead to permanent sterilization. That means they will never be able to impregnate women in the future.

What is not clear yet is evidence about how sperm exposed to radiation affects children made from the sperm (NCI, 2022). It is also noted that some men whose prostate gland is exposed to radiation may become impotent or may not be able to have an erection. From experience, older men don't care about the side effects that affect their sexuality compared to younger males. On the other hand, men of African descent of all ages have a bigger concern with their sexuality than other ethnic groups. As always, these concerns should be raised to your healthcare team, who, among other recommendations, will advise men who wish to have children in the future to store their sperm in the sperm bank.

Sex

Most patients who are going through radiation therapy don't have the desire for any sexual intercourse at this point. Again, everybody is different. When radiation treatment involves the pelvic and sex organs, people may notice changes in their ability to enjoy sex. In some situations, the level of desire decreases.

Women: When women are being radiated in their pelvic area, they are advised not to have sex. The reason is that it might be very painful. Treatment in this area may also cause vaginal dryness, itching and burning. These are short-term effects that will subside a couple of weeks after treatment, and the patient will be able to go about their sex life. On the contrary, there might be long-term effects, such as scars, which could affect vaginal stretchability during sex. This may sometimes cause problems in marital homes, especially among young couples. I have had situations where some men have divorced their wives because they can't have sex with them. To satisfy their sexual desire, it is not unusual for some men to have extramarital affairs.

Men: Sometimes, radiation treatment will affect the nerves that allow a man to have an erection. For those who are facing this problem, it does occur gradually over many months or years. I remember talking to one of my former male patients about sex. He told me he had been having regular sex for years but that it depended on the position he found with his wife. Couples are advised to talk about their sex lives, for it could be some good therapy. Again, your healthcare team is a good resource for consultation. In extreme circumstances, expert sex therapeutic services might be needed.

Emotions

Nobody wants to be sick or go to the hospital. It makes matters worse when a person has cancer, which is a life-threatening disease. The fact that someone has been diagnosed with the disease is enough to evoke anger, fear, anxiety, depression, a sense of helplessness, fatigue from the radiation, and even the constant movement to and from the hospital is emotionally draining.

Now, note that whatever emotional pain a patient might be experiencing is only temporal. It will be over immediately after treatment is complete or a couple of weeks after completion. On the other hand, patients are advised to join a support group. This is because most people in this group are either in your position or have been in your situation.

Heart Complications

Patients who are having radiation treatment around the chest area have a likelihood of having heart complications or a risk of heart disease (NCI, 2022). This risk increases with higher doses of radiation and a larger treatment area. This is equally noticeable with patients who have their left breast and the side of their lungs treated with radiation. It is also noted that radiation can cause heart valve damage, irregular heartbeats, and sometimes hardening of the arteries, which makes it more likely for future heart attacks (NCI, 2022).

Radiation Pneumonitis

Radiation pneumonitis is the inflammation of the lungs that comes about because of radiation treatment to the chest area. It is noted to occur about 3 to 6 months after the initial radiation treatment (ACS, 2019). Studies show that it is more likely to occur if a patient has other lung diseases like emphysema. Some more symptoms of pneumonitis include cough, weakness, low-grade fever, pink-tinged sputum, shortness of breath that gets worse with exercise, and chest pain that gets worse when a patient is taking a deep breath.

It is also noted that with radiation pneumonitis, sometimes there are no symptoms, and it can only be found after taking a chest X-ray. If there are symptoms, as severe as they may be, they will often go away on their own. On the other hand, if treatment is needed, it is only to decrease inflammation, and most people will recover without any long-lasting effects (ACS, 2019). If, for some reason, it persists, it may lead to stiffening and scarring of the lungs, a condition known as pulmonary fibrosis. In such a situation, the lungs can no longer fully inflate and take in air.

Questions for your Doctor

1. What type of radiation therapy treatment am I getting?

2. Why am I getting radiation therapy and not another form of treatment for my cancer?

3. What happens if I don't get radiation therapy for my cancer?

4. What does radiation do to cancer?

5. When and how do I find out if the treatment is effective or not?

6. Do I have other treatment options than radiation therapy?

7. Will I be radioactive while having radiation therapy?

8. What are the short- and long-term side effects of the radiation?

9. Are there special precautions during and after treatment?

10. Are there any eating restrictions while on treatment?

11. What are the consequences of skipping some treatments?

12. What is the duration of my treatment?

13. Will I be able to undertake my daily activities while undergoing radiation therapy treatment?

14. What should I do to get ready for radiation treatment?

15. How many patients with my type of cancer have you treated so far?

16. Can I eat before my treatment?

References

1. Cure. Combining Science and Humanity. Cancer Updates, Research and Education: www.CURETODAY.COM

2. Chen, H., Collins, A. R., Conell, M., Damia, G., Dasgupta, S., Ferguson, L. R. et al. (December 2015). "Genomic instability in human cancer: Molecular insights and opportunities for therapeutic attack and prevention through diet and nutrition" (https://www.ncbi.nim.nih.gov/pmc/articles/PMC4600419).

3. Murphy, G.P., Morris, L.B., & Lange, D. Informed Decisions. The Complete Book of Cancer Diagnosis, Treatment, and Recovery. American Cancer Society. Pub. VIKING 1997.

4. Weiss, M.C. & Weiss, E. (1997, 1998). Living Beyond Breast Cancer. A Survivor's Guide for When Treatment Ends and the Rest of Your Life Begins. Times Books.

5. National Cancer Institute. Clinical Trials Information for Patients and Caregivers. Cancer.gov. https://www.cancer.gov/about-cancer/treatment/clinical-research-trials-you. Reviewed February 6/2020. Accessed July 29/2020.

6. Patient Empowerment Network. https://powerful patients.org/2019/08/06/will-cancer-be-cured-by-2020/

7. Springer-Verlag. Cancer in Children. Clinical Management. Berlin Heidelberg New York 1975.

8. US Department of Health and Human Services. Preventing Tobacco Use Among Youth and Young Adults: A Report of the Surgeon General. 2012. Accessed at https://www.ncbi.nlm.nih.gov/books/NBK99237/ on October 5.2020.

9. Vladimir Lange, M.D. Be a Survivor. Colorectal Cancer Treatment Guide. Roche Pharmaceuticals. www.langeproductions.com

Index